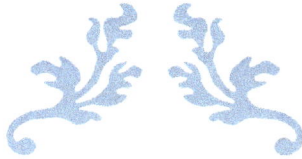

CURB YOUR APPETITE NATURALLY FOR LASTING WEIGHT LOSS

The Satiety Starter

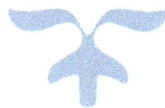

By Hester Y Cheong

Cover design and layout by: Yoke Yin CHEONG

First Kindle edition, 2025

For permissions, inquiries, or feedback, contact:

cheong.hester@gmail.com

ISBNs

eBook: 978-0-473-74774-9

Paperback: 978-0-473-74772-5

Hardcover: 978-0-473-74773-2

Contents

"I did the research so you would not have to chew through all the journals. Let us begin...."

— Hester Y Cheong

Opening Insights

In today's world, **being slim is often equated with beauty**. At the same time, the medical community stresses the importance of maintaining a healthy weight to lower the risk of heart disease, diabetes, and other chronic conditions. People invest staggering amounts of time, effort, and money in the pursuit of weight loss. Yet for many, the journey feels like an uphill battle— some struggle to lose any weight at all, while others regain it in half the time it took to lose it.

Weight gain is shaped by a **complex interplay of genetics, lifestyle, and our modern food environment**. Our genes influence how effectively we regulate appetite, and intriguingly, the human body is designed to defend energy stores—a biological legacy from times when food was scarce and fat storage was essential for survival.

But today, the situation has flipped. Food is **plentiful and constantly accessible**, while modern life encourages **sedentary behaviour**. This clash between ancient biology and contemporary convenience makes weight gain feel almost inevitable.

Are we destined to become overweight? Absolutely not.

While our biology may incline us to store energy, we are not powerless. With a deeper understanding of how appetite works, we can make smarter choices and take control of our health.

The key to sustainable weight management lies in **understanding why we overeat**. Research shows that individuals prone to weight gain often experience a **delayed satiety response**—they eat more before they begin to feel full. Satiety is that internal signal of fullness that tells you to stop eating. If overeating is driven by a delay in this response, could there be a simple way to eat less—without resorting to extreme diets, medications, or surgery?

The answer lies in **scientifically designed starters**, or "**preloads**" as they are commonly referred to in research. With the right composition and timing, these small appetizers can help you feel full faster and **naturally reduce**

overall food intake. Once you understand the principles behind these preloads, you can easily prepare these starters yourself and fit them into your everyday routine.

We have all seen diet trends come and go—some may bring quick results by cutting out an entire macronutrient. And yes, the weight may come off at first—but not because of magic. It is simply a result of reduced calorie intake. The challenge begins when the body adjusts, and people compensate by eating more of other macronutrients. Progress stalls, balance slips, and the weight often returns—in half the time it took to lose it.

The same goes for fasting which has gained popularity in recent years. While rooted in religious and cultural traditions and possibly beneficial for some, its success depends entirely on how it is practiced. Fasting reduces meal frequency, which may lower calorie intake—but if followed by binge eating during post-fast, the benefits are quickly undone. In some cases, it may even lead to rebound weight gain. I have seen this happen firsthand. It is a reminder that **consistency and balance are more powerful than extremes**.

Low-carb, keto, or fasting plans may offer benefits for those managing diabetes or pre-diabetes, such as improved blood glucose and insulin sensitivity—but those benefits are condition-specific.

Of course, if you have found a dietary approach that works for you—one that fits your goals and lifestyle—then stick with it. As the saying goes, *different strokes for different folks*.

That said, one of the hardest parts of maintaining any diet is managing hunger and preventing overeating. That is where this strategy fits in. Whether you follow fasting, keto, low-carb, Mediterranean, or a flexible approach, **controlling food volume and energy density is key**. And if you do fast, avoiding post-fast binge eating is crucial to lasting success.

That is exactly the reason what you are about to discover in this Book matters.

This Book grew out of my Master's research in Exercise and Nutrition Science at the University of Chester (UK), where I graduated with Distinction. Since then, new studies have continued to support the approach I share here. I have updated the content with the latest science—translating complex research into clear, practical strategies that are easy to understand and apply.

After countless hours of research and writing, I am excited to share these tools to help you take control of your appetite and create lasting change. Knowledge should not sit unused—it should drive real results. That is why I have made this Book both accessible and affordable for anyone ready to improve their health.

An Important Guide to Terms Used in This Book

Before we dive in, here is a brief overview of key terms and abbreviations used throughout this Book. Understanding them will help you get the most out of the content ahead.

Satiety is the feeling of fullness and satisfaction that signals you to stop eating. It helps regulate how much food you consume by reducing hunger after a meal.

Preload vs Starter. In most nutritional research, a *preload* refers to a small amount of food or drink consumed shortly before a meal, typically in a controlled study, to examine how specific food properties (like energy density, macronutrient composition, or volume) affect appetite, satiety, and energy intake.

A pre-meal **starter (British) or an appetizer (American)** in this Book— is a practical, application of the preload concept. It involves consuming a small, strategic portion of food or drink—such as a soup, salad, or piece of fruit—shortly before the main meal. It gently activates the body's natural satiety signals, helps you feel fuller sooner and reduces overeating. The term **"satiety starter"** I use later in this Book perfectly captures the essence of the concept—it combines the **timing** (a starter) and the **purpose** (to boost satiety) in a way that is both simple and intuitive.

In this Book, "preload" is used in research contexts, while "satiety starter" is a term I use when those findings are translated into practical, everyday recipes.

Test meal. In research studies, a **test meal** refers to the main meal consumed after a preload, typically used to measure subsequent food intake and satiety—comparable to a main course in a typical eating occasion.

BMI (Body Mass Index) To better understand the studies ahead, let me clarify BMI (Body Mass Index). BMI is calculated as:

$$BMI = weight\ (kg) \div height^2\ (m^2)$$

A **healthy BMI** generally falls between **18.5 and 25**. The healthy BMI range must be taken in context with the person's physical activity levels. For example, endurance athletes may have lower BMI while bodybuilders may have a higher BMI.

A **BMI of under 21** often reflects a naturally **lean body** type. In this range, further weight loss may not be necessary or beneficial. Instead, focus on a **balanced, nutrient-rich diet**—plenty of vegetables, fruits, lean protein-rich foods, moderate healthy carbs and small amount of healthy fats—alongside **regular physical activity** to support overall well-being.

If your BMI falls **below 18.5**, it indicates you are already on the lighter side. If you still feel the **urge to lose weight**, I strongly recommend consulting a **registered dietitian** for personalised guidance to ensure your nutritional needs are fully supported.

Body fat composition: While BMI correlates well with body fat, it is only a general indicator. **Body composition tools** like smartwatches and bioelectrical impedance devices offer more precise data by measuring both **fat and lean mass**.

Ideal **body fat percentages** are:

- **Men:** 12%–20%

- **Women:** 21%–32%

These insights help provide a clearer picture of overall health beyond just weight or BMI alone. Again, context of physical activities matters - long distance runner and aerobic exercise professionals may have fat mass as low as 3%.

et al. is an abbreviation of the Latin phrase *et alia*, which means "and others."

It is commonly used in academic writing when referring to a study or paper with multiple authors. Instead of listing all the authors' names, only the first author's name is mentioned, followed by *et al.* to represent the rest. This keeps references concise and readable, especially when citing studies with many contributors.

Examples: Instead of writing: *Smith, Johnson, Lee, and Patel (2020)*, I write: *Smith et al. (2020)*

Statistically significant means the result of a study is unlikely to be due to chance. In research, this signals that the effect observed is probably real, not accidental.

Scientists often compare two groups—for example, one given a drink before a meal and one without. If there is a noticeable difference, they run statistical calculations to see if it is likely genuine. If the numbers say it is highly unlikely to be random, the result is said to be **statistically significant** or there is a **significant difference.**

In this Book, think of statistical significance as meaning **important, meaningful, or** simply that **the result matters.**

kcal and Calories mean the same thing on food labels. Technically, 1 kcal = 1 Calorie = 1,000 small calories—but in nutrition, we just say "calories" for short. Some countries use **kilojoules (kJ)** instead. To convert:

- **kJ → kcal: divide by 4.184**

- **kcal → kJ: multiply by 4.184**

So, if a label shows energy in kJ, just divide to get the calorie value you want to compare it with. In the food tables in Appendix B, I have provided both values. Calories (kcal) and kJ are measures of energy which are stored in the human body as fats.

1 The Inspiration and Aim of This Book

Recent research has revealed something powerful that overwrites attempts to lose weight. Our body weight is not just the result of willpower—it is biologically regulated, with genetics setting a kind of internal "set point." The body resists change through hormonal and neural signals that drive appetite and protect fat stores. This is why many traditional weight-loss methods fail in the long run.

Additionally, as we age, our **metabolic rate naturally declines**, largely due to a gradual loss of muscle mass—which means we burn fewer calories at rest. At the same time, our body's **appetite suppression mechanisms may weaken**, with satiety signals becoming slower or less effective. Burning less energy while feeling less full—can quietly shift the energy balance toward weight gain and drive the "set-point" up.

Even pharmaceutical approaches often trigger counteractive responses in other pathways, making sustainable weight loss even more difficult. But does that mean any weight loss is hopeless? Of course not.

The real challenge lies in the approach. Diets are notoriously difficult to maintain (Freedman, 2001), and have shown inconsistent results. Most diets focus on cutting things out—carbs, fat, entire meals —rather than understanding how our body decides *when* and *how much* to eat. Satiety, the body's natural fullness signal, holds the key. When we work with it, not against it, we gain a sustainable edge.

This Book presents a smarter, science-based strategy: using a simple, targeted **pre-meal**—which I called a **satiety starter (or appetizer)**—to naturally boost fullness and reduce calorie intake. No extreme diets. No starvation. Just a practical, research-backed way to regain control—by **harnessing your body's own biology**.

1.1 Why Focus on Preloads?

Instead of battling hunger with willpower alone or relying on restrictive diets, preloads offer a smarter, science-backed solution. Research into satiety, macronutrients, and eating behaviour shows that preloading—having a small, targeted portion of food before your main meal—can naturally curb appetite and reduce calorie intake without side effects.

Extensive research has been conducted on appetite control, satiety, macronutrient composition, and behavioral differences in eating habits. However, among the many methods explored, **preloading appears to be a promising, repeatable, and side-effect-free strategy for reducing calorie intake.**

If overeating is driven by a delayed satiety response, then consuming the right preload at the right time could help moderate food intake in individuals struggling with weight gain. Preloads may offer short-term satiety benefits and, when used consistently, could provide **a sustainable, drug-free way to manage energy intake**.

1.2 The Approach of This Book

Rather than adding another single preload study to the growing body of research on preloads, this Book **takes a systematic review approach**—analysing and compiling findings from numerous studies to create a clear and comprehensive picture of how preloading influences appetite and energy intake.

Many studies confirm that **preloads reduce food intake in the meal** that follows, but results vary when looking at overall energy balance. This Book aims to identify the **optimal preload strategy**—the composition, timing, and conditions that lead to meaningful reductions in calorie consumption.

By bringing together the latest scientific insights, this Book provides practical guidance on **how to use preloads effectively** to support appetite control and sustainable weight management—without relying on willpower alone.

1.3 A Practical Guide to Effective Preloading

This Book presents a clear, science-backed model for using preloads to naturally reduce calorie intake and curb overeating. By analyzing findings from existing studies, it uncovers the key factors that make preloading most effective, including:

✅ The best macronutrient composition – Which nutrients help you feel fuller, longer?

✅ Ideal energy levels – How much is just enough to curb appetite without adding excess calories?

✅ Optimal portion size – Should preloads be light or more substantial?

✅ Timing matters – When is the best time to consume a preload for maximum impact?

✅ Solid vs. liquid – Does texture and form affect satiety?

✅ Individual differences – How do preloads work for different people?

By breaking down these factors, this Book provides a practical, easy-to-follow guide on how to use preloads effectively—helping you take control of your appetite and achieve sustainable weight management!

This Book is based on a **Master's dissertation in Exercise and Nutrition Science** submitted to the University of Chester. The original research followed a **systematic review approach**, carefully analysing existing studies on preloading and appetite control.

To keep the content **up-to-date and relevant**, newer research findings have been incorporated, ensuring you get the most current insights backed by science.

For those who love the details, the full research methodology is outlined in Appendix A. But if you are just here for the practical takeaways—feel free to move onto the content that follows!

2 The Bigger Picture

Let us zoom out and take a look at the bigger picture first, so you can truly grasp the factors fueling the global obesity epidemic. Once we have that foundation, we will dive into the heart of the issue and explore how we can tackle the delay in the feeling of fullness—one of the key drivers behind overeating.

2.1 The Global Obesity Crisis: A Battle That is Here to Stay

Obesity has been declared a **global epidemic** by the World Health Organization as early as 1998 (WHO, 1998). But unlike 'short-term' health crises such as COVID-19, obesity is not going away. According to statistics released by WHO (2024), over one billion people aged 5 years and older worldwide are living with obesity.

In 2018, it is reported that nearly 20% of children and over 40% of adults in the United States were considered obese with the adult rate of obesity predicted to rise to 50% by 2030 (Szalanczy et al. 2018).

"Overweight and obesity have reached epidemic proportions in the WHO European Region, affecting almost 60% of adults. ... Alarmingly, there have been consistent increases in the prevalence of overweight and obesity in the WHO European Region and no Member State is on track to reach the target of halting the rise in obesity by 2025." (WHO, 2022).

What is even more alarming is that this surge is not confined to wealthier nations; many **newly industrialized countries** have transitioned from battling malnutrition to struggling with rising obesity rates.

Repeating, if you are **struggling with your weight**, you are **NOT alone**.

2.2 It is not only a "Calories In, Calories Out" equation

While energy balance still matters, the old belief that weight is simply a matter of calories in versus calories out has evolved into something far more complex. Research shows that our bodies defend a **stable weight "set point"** — our body built-in mechanism resists short-term weight changes (Kassirer & Angell, 1998). Unfortunately, for many of us, this set point tends to **creep upward** over time, especially as **metabolism slows** and **physical activity declines** with age.

Feedback loops in the central nervous system tightly regulate appetite and metabolism to maintain this set point. Though extreme dieting and intense exercise can temporarily push the system, the body often **rebounds** the moment those efforts stop, fighting to restore its original weight. This explains why **sustained weight loss** often feels like an uphill battle.

Adding to the challenge, research has revealed a strong **genetic influence** on weight regulation (Aitman, 2003; Lindpaintner, 1995). Some individuals are biologically **programmed to struggle** with weight control. Obesity is not just about willpower — it is the result of a complex dance between **genes, environment, lifestyle**, and **biology**. For many, managing weight is not simply about making better choices; it is about working against powerful internal systems designed to protect body fat.

2.4 Key Research Findings on Obesity and Weight Regulation

Over the years, scientific research has uncovered several critical insights into obesity and weight management. Here are some of the most important findings:

o **Metabolism is not to blame:** Contrary to popular belief, obesity is not caused by a slower metabolism. Instead, it is primarily driven by consuming more energy than the body needs (Stensel et al., 2001).

o **Energy imbalance fuels weight gain:** Modern lifestyles have become increasingly sedentary, yet food intake has not decreased to match this lower energy expenditure. This disconnect between diet and activity levels has significantly contributed to rising obesity rates (Prentice & Jebb, 1995; Lahti-Koski et al., 2002).

o **Genetics play a major role:** Individual genetic predisposition affects weight control, influencing how the body stores fat, regulates hunger, and responds to food intake (Lindpainter, 1995; Ristow et al., 1998).

o **Physiology drives eating behavior:** These genetic differences manifest in physiological responses to food, affecting appetite, satiety signals, and overall eating patterns (Korner et al., 2003).

o **Delayed satiety leads to overeating:** Studies have found that individuals prone to weight gain tend to eat larger portions and take longer to feel full compared to weight-stable individuals. This delayed satiety response encourages overeating (Pearcey & Castro, 2002).

o **Weight has a natural "set point":** A person's weight appears to have a biological set point—a range the body naturally resists moving beyond, whether through weight loss or gain (Pearcey & Castro, 2002). However, this set point may shift with age.

o **Appetite regulation is complex:** Hunger and satiety are governed by intricate interactions between gastrointestinal hormones and macronutrient metabolism. Each nutrient type follows its own metabolic cycle, influencing when and how much we eat (Read et al., 1994; Korner et al., 2003; Szalanczy et al., 2022)

2.5   The Secrets of Metabolism

Forget the myth: overweight and obese individuals do not struggle with weight because of a "slow metabolism." In a study comparing 20 obese and 20 non-obese Singaporean boys (of Chinese descent), Stensel et al. (2001) found that in absolute terms, **obese boys actually had a slightly higher resting metabolic rate (RMR)** than their non-obese peers (see Figure 1).

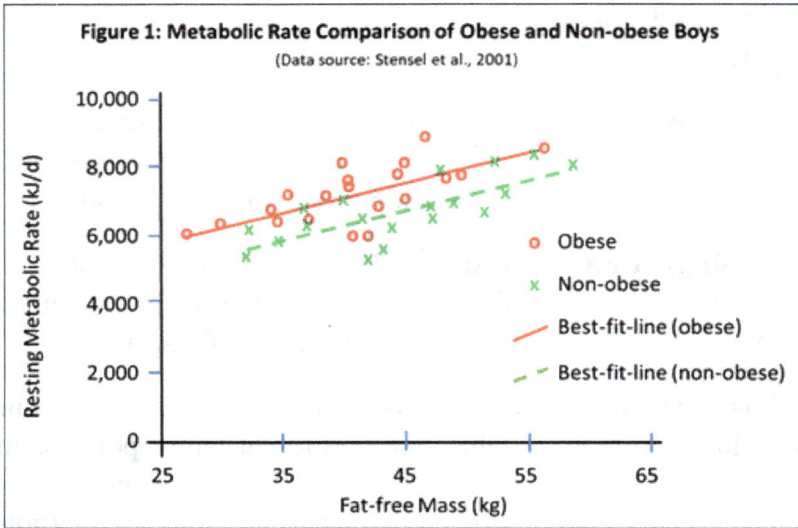

Figure 1: Metabolic Rate Comparison of Obese and Non-obese Boys
(Data source: Stensel et al., 2001)

This research clearly **debunks the old belief** that obesity stems from a sluggish metabolism. The real driver of weight gain is **excess calorie intake or lack of physical activities—not a lower-than-normal metabolism.**

(This is not to be confused with age-related metabolic slow-down.)

2.6   *The Sedentary Trap*

Obesity has been a growing problem in developed countries for decades, fueled not only by diet, but by increasingly **sedentary lifestyles**.

2.6.1 Secular Modern Conveniences and Obesity

Prentice and Jebb (1995) found a striking link: as **car and television ownership** rose, so did obesity rates, even though **fat intake and total calorie intake** in Britain had declined between 1970 to1990. Their findings highlight a key paradox — it is not just what we eat, but how little we move that drives the obesity epidemic. The data make it clear: **modern**

conveniences have reshaped daily life at the cost of physical activity. (As illustrated in Figure 2.)

As people become more sedentary—spending more time in cars and in front of screens—**obesity rates continue to climb**. While this study is based on population trends and should be interpreted with caution, it underscores a crucial point: **low physical activity significantly contributes to weight gain by reducing energy expenditure**.

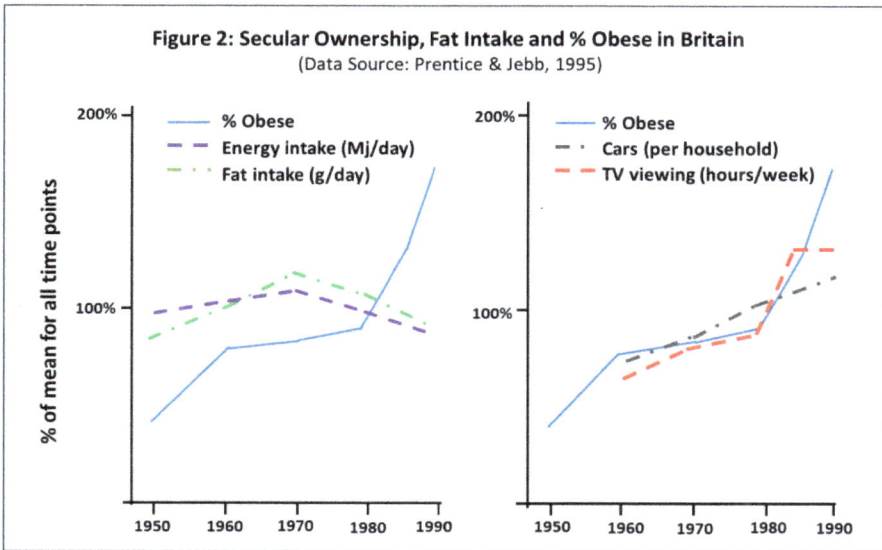

Figure 2: Secular Ownership, Fat Intake and % Obese in Britain
(Data Source: Prentice & Jebb, 1995)

In today's digital world, where social interactions and information searches happen online rather than through physical activity, **the challenge of obesity persists**. A study of 1,060 Health Sciences students at Simón Bolívar University found that **smartphone use over five hours a day** raised the **risk of obesity by 43%**. Heavy users were **twice as likely** to consume sugary drinks, fast food, and snacks, and were less active. (Accinelli et al., 2019)

A national study of nearly 30,000 U.S. adolescents found that just **over an hour a day** of TV or video games raised the risk of overweight and obesity by **40%**, while **4 or more hours** more than **doubled** it. Heavy use of handheld devices also increased risk, but to a lesser extent. Regular exercise helped protect against weight gain, while **inactivity made screen time's impact worse** — with girls showing greater vulnerability than boys. (Bakour et al., 2022)

2.6.2 Leisure-Time Physical Activity

Lahti-Koski et al. (2002) found a strong link between leisure-time physical activity and lower BMI. Over 15 years, they tracked more than 24,000 Finnish men and women and observed that those who were more active during their free time consistently had lower BMIs and a lower risk of obesity.

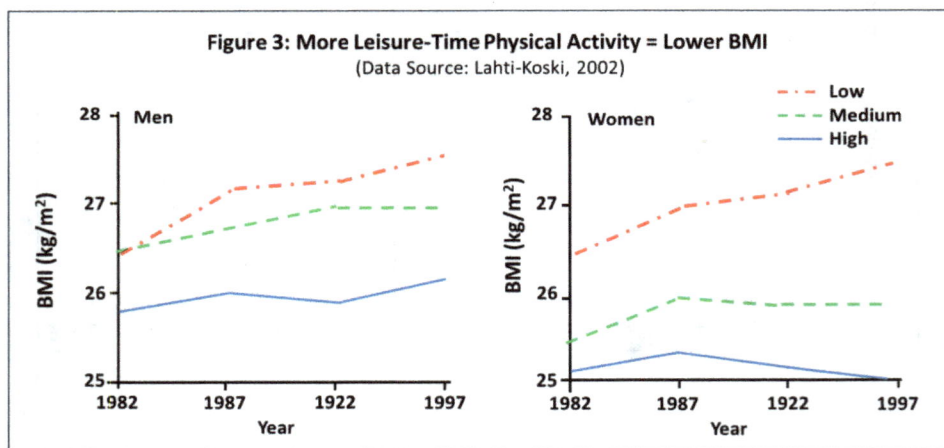

Figure 3: More Leisure-Time Physical Activity = Lower BMI
(Data Source: Lahti-Koski, 2002)

As shown in Figure 3, the trend was clear: the more people moved, the healthier their weight. Those with little to no leisure-time physical activity saw the biggest BMI increases, reinforcing how regular physical activity can help maintain a healthy weight and reduce obesity risk.

The link between leisure-time activity and lower BMI grew even stronger over time—especially in women. As leisure-time exercise increased, both BMI and obesity rates declined.

This trend highlights just how important regular physical activity is for maintaining a healthy weight and reducing the risk of obesity.

2.6.3 Jobs and Obesity

The Lahti-Koski et al. (2002) study also found clear links between job type and BMI over 15 years. Men who were not working had the greatest BMI increases, while those in physically demanding jobs consistently had the lowest. A similar pattern was seen in women—those not working had the highest BMI across the years. See Figure 4 for details.

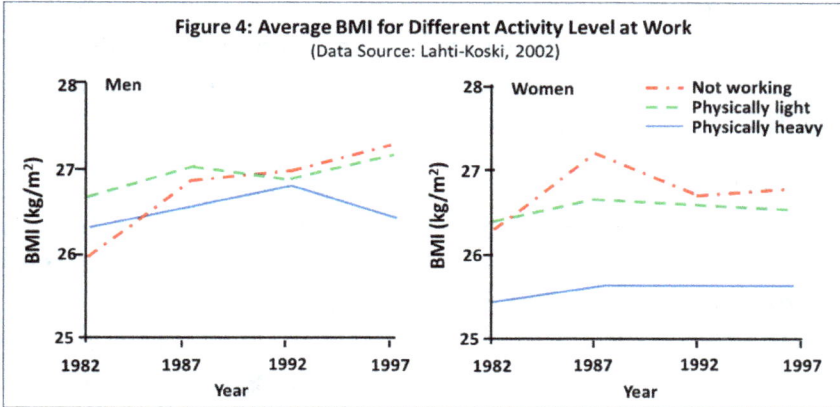

Figure 4: Average BMI for Different Activity Level at Work
(Data Source: Lahti-Koski, 2002)

This underscores the role of everyday physical activity—both at work and during free time—in preventing weight gain and supporting a healthy body weight.

2.7 *The Growing Imbalance behind Weight Gain - Eating Outpaces Physical Activities –*

The McCrory et al. (2002) study highlights a worrying trend in the U.S.: while physical activity levels stayed roughly the same from 1990 to 1998, average daily calorie intake jumped by 340 kcal between 1984 and 1994. This widening gap—**eating more without moving more**—helps explain why people are **gaining weight younger and faster**.

The study also points to subtle yet powerful influences on eating habits, like oversized portions, snacking, eating out, liquid calories, and highly tempting foods. Over time, these habits quietly push people toward overeating.

As our bodies do not automatically adjust food intake when we burn fewer calories, this mismatch between intake and energy use plays a key role in rising obesity rates.

2.8   *How a Slower Satiety Response Fuels Overeating*

Satiety—the signal that tells us to stop eating—does not arrive at the same time for everyone. For some, it lags behind, causing them to keep eating long after their body has had enough. This delay, influenced by hormones, metabolism, and even the type of food eaten, can silently fuel weight gain.

Pearcey and Castro (2002) revealed this in a fascinating study: **people who were gaining weight ate larger meals than those who maintained their weight, even though both groups had similar lifestyles and meal frequencies.** The key difference? The weight-gaining group simply did not stop eating when the normal weight-stable group had. They averaged 380 extra kcal (1,600 kJ) a day—enough to add 16 kg (35 lbs) of fat in a year—yet they did not feel hungrier or more satisfied than others. It was not willpower, but biology.

What about diet composition? The weight-gaining individuals ate more fat, but that was not the main culprit—it was simply the total amount of food consumed. Eating in social settings also did not explain the larger portions, and emotional factors, while potentially influential, did not show a significant impact in this study.

Why This Matters?

Further supporting this, Llewellyn et al. (2013) found that some people are genetically predisposed to feel full more slowly. In a world full of tempting, high-calorie foods, this makes it dangerously easy to overeat. Recognising delayed satiety as a physiological trait—not a personal failing—is essential. It also explains why strategies like pre-meal "satiety starters" can help: they give your body a head-start on feeling full, curbing overeating before it begins.

In ancient times, when generations repeatedly succumbed to the same illness, it was often believed to be a family curse—an ominous force passed down through the bloodline. In reality, what was at work was not a supernatural curse but genetics. Traits inherited from one generation to the next unknowingly perpetuated diseases, making it seem as though families were doomed by fate.

Obesity, much like other inherited conditions, is shaped by a complex interplay of genetics, lifestyle, and environment. While diet and exercise are key contributors, genetic factors heavily influence how the body stores fat, regulates appetite, and burns calories.

Some people struggle with weight due to **rare** *monogenic mutations* where a **single faulty gene** leads to **severe, early-onset obesity**. These genes play critical roles in regulating hunger and satiety. When disrupted, they impair the body's ability to sense fullness, causing a stronger drive to eat before feeling satisfied. Many monogenic genes had been discovered.   Some examples include:

- **MC4R (Melanocortin 4 Receptor):** Mutations in the MC4R gene impair the brain's ability to detect signals from leptin and insulin to regulate hunger and energy balance, leading to excessive appetite and weight gain. This is one of the most common genetic causes of severe, early-onset obesity.

- **LEP (Leptin):** Leptin is produced by adipose tissues. Mutations in the LEP gene result in leptin deficiency. The brain perceives the low leptin level as starvation, which leads to increased appetite and reduced energy expenditure.

- **LEPR (Leptin Receptor):** Dysfunctional LEPR prevents leptin from binding to its receptor in the brain, disrupting appetite regulation and causing persistent hunger, leading to early-onset obesity.

- **POMC (Pro-opiomelanocortin):** Mutations in the POMC gene impair the production of the alpha-MSH hormone, which normally suppresses appetite, leading to severe hyperphagia and early obesity.

- **GHRL (Ghrelin):** Variations in the GHRL gene can increase ghrelin levels, promoting hunger and reduced satiety, which contributes to excessive eating and early weight gain.

More commonly, people carry a mix of low-risk genes, for example the FTO (fat mass and obesity) variant, that subtly nudge them toward bigger appetites and cravings for calorie-dense foods. Variants of FTO are linked to stronger hunger signals and cravings for high-calorie foods, which can make resisting temptation much harder.

This **polygenic pattern** means dozens, even hundreds, of small genetic variations each nudge the body toward gaining weight. According to Szalanczy et al., 2022 there are more than **900 known** low-risk common **genetic variants** associated with body mass index (BMI).

These **genetic traits often run in families**, helping explain why obesity tends to cluster within households. Genes not only influence appetite and satiety but also affect where fat is stored—some individuals are genetically predisposed to carry more weight around the waist, increasing the risk of heart disease and type 2 diabetes.

However, the sharp rise in obesity rates over the past few decades cannot be blamed on genetics alone—our DNA has remained largely unchanged. Instead, modern lifestyles have created an environment that promotes weight gain: more time spent sitting, increased reliance on cars, and constant exposure to energy-dense, highly palatable foods.

People respond differently to this environment. Due to genetic variation, some are more susceptible to gaining weight, while others remain stable even under similar conditions. This highlights just how complex the interaction between genes and environment truly is.

2.10   Appetite Control - How the Body Regulates Food Intake

The human body naturally supports a routine of three to four meals per day, with physiological systems playing a key role in regulating hunger and fullness. Internal mechanisms largely determine when we start and stop eating.

One of the quickest signals of fullness is **gastric distension**—the stomach expanding as we eat—but this **effect is temporary**. Interestingly, when food reaches the small intestine, it activates chemoreceptors that slow digestion, enhance satiety, and reduce food intake.

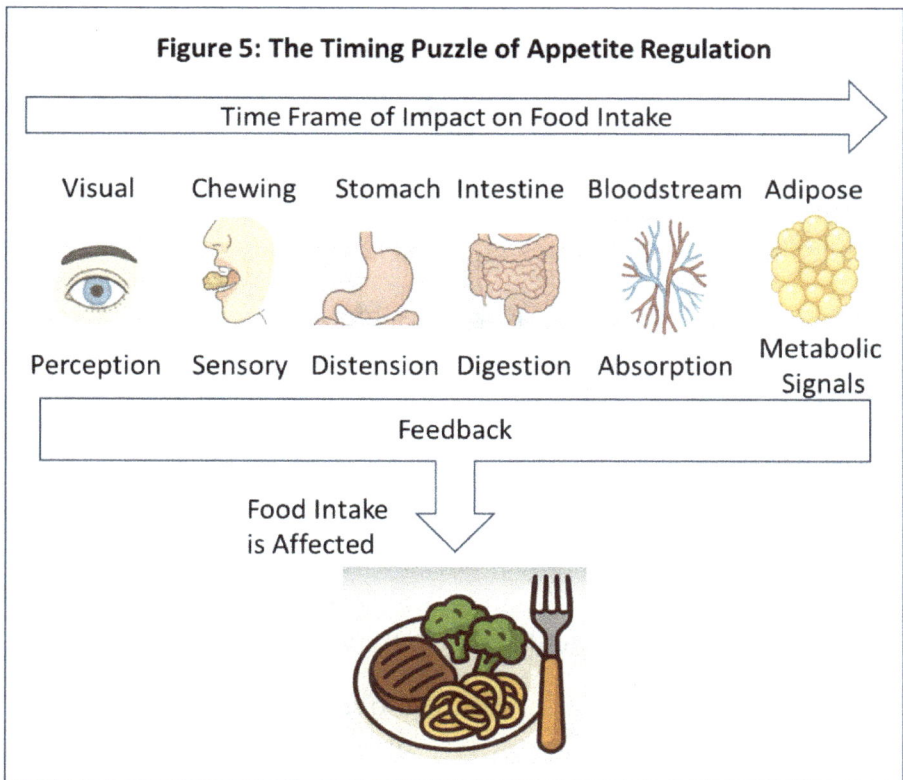

Figure 5: The Timing Puzzle of Appetite Regulation

Our bodies use a complex feedback system to regulate food intake. Our food intake is influenced by various levels of feedback (Benelam, 2009) as illustrated in Figure 5 and simplified below:

- o **Cognitive Phase** begins before the first bite, influenced by expectations, memories, and visual appearance. The brain anticipates food intake and stimulates the appetite.

- o **Sensory cues** from taste, texture and chewing. The tastier the food, the more a person eats.

- o **Gastric Phase** starts when food reaches the stomach. Stomach stretching sends signals to the brain, transient but crucial in meal termination.

- o **Intestinal Phase** Digestion continues in the intestines, gut hormones like GLP-1, PYY, and CCK are released. These hormones enhance the feeling of fullness and slow down eating.

- o **Absorption Phase:** Nutrients absorbed into the bloodstream are detected by receptors in the body and brain. These receptors influence ongoing satiety — how long fullness lasts after a meal.

- o **Metabolic Signalling:** Hormones like leptin provide the brain with information about fat stores. Help regulate appetite and food intake over time.

In simple terms, the mouth and gut decide when and how much we eat in the moment, while metabolic signals manage long-term energy balance. These different phases vary in effectiveness in different individuals, giving rise to different responses and different ability to manage one's weight.

Energy requirements and food intake are also shaped by a mix of physiological and cognitive influences. Factors like pregnancy, lactation, growth and physical activity increase the body's metabolic demand. While mood, mental focus, and the social environment affect eating behaviour through psychological pathways. Together, these elements drive both how much energy the body needs and how much food we consume.

2.11 How Appetite-Regulating Hormones Influence Food Intake?

Beyond meal-to-meal signals, the digestive system adapts over time. While the stomach does not permanently shrink or grow based on eating habits, receptors in the small intestine adjust to nutrient levels, affecting digestion and absorption. Key hormones like insulin, cortisol, and thyroid hormone further influence this process, with factors like obesity, pregnancy, and illness triggering additional changes.

The brain, particularly the hypothalamus, acts as a command centre for balancing energy intake and expenditure. Specialized sensors in the gut, liver, and brain continuously monitor nutrient levels, adjusting hunger and satiety signals to maintain energy balance. The hunger and fullness regulation system are a complex one. When this system is disrupted, it can contribute to overeating and weight gain.

Although psychosocial factors play a role in eating behaviour, the physiological control of food intake appears to be mediated in part by various gastrointestinal mechanisms that trigger both the initiation and termination of eating behaviours. (Figure 6)

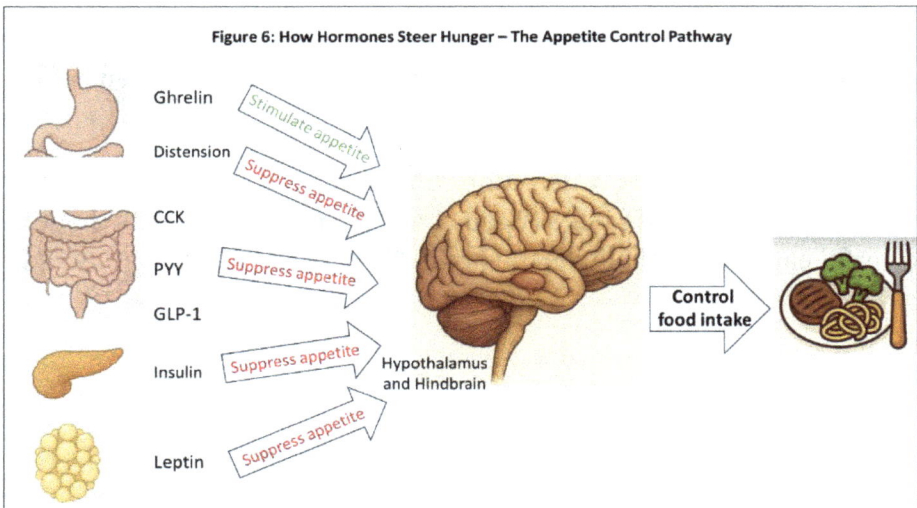

Figure 6: How Hormones Steer Hunger – The Appetite Control Pathway

- ### Ghrelin – The Hunger Hormone

Ghrelin is the only known **orexigenic** (appetite-stimulating) hormone and is secreted primarily from the **stomach** when it is empty.

Its effects:

- Activates **NPY/AgRP neurons** in the **hypothalamus**, triggering hunger.

- Stimulates **food-seeking behaviour** and increases meal size.

Ghrelin peaks before meals and falls quickly after eating—unless overridden by other hormones like PYY or GLP-1.

- ### Cholecystokinin (CCK) – The Early Satiety Signal

CCK is one of the first hormones to respond when food enters the small intestine—especially fats and proteins. It is secreted by cells in the **duodenum** (the first section of the small intestine). Once released, CCK performs a dual role:

- **Digestive support:** It stimulates the **gallbladder** to release bile and the **pancreas** to secrete digestive enzymes.

- **Appetite suppression:** It sends a satiety signal via the **vagus nerve** to the **hypothalamus**, helping to curb hunger even before the meal ends.

Even **low doses of CCK**, when infused intravenously, have been shown to significantly reduce food intake (Read et al., 1994). This suggests that CCK is a powerful early signal that tells the brain, "You've had enough."

- ## GLP-1 (Glucagon-Like Peptide-1) – The Blood Sugar & Satiety Booster

As food travels further into the **ileum and colon**, **GLP-1** is secreted by **L-cells** in response to nutrient absorption. Its key roles

- Boosts **insulin** release and suppresses **glucagon**, helping regulate blood sugar.

- **Slows stomach emptying**, which keeps you feeling full longer.

- **Enhances satiety signals** to the brain, reducing appetite and food intake.

Because of these powerful effects, GLP-1 has become the basis for several possible obesity and type 2 diabetes treatments.

- ## Peptide YY (PYY) – The Long-Lasting Appetite Brake

PYY is also secreted by **L-cells** in the **small intestine and colon**, usually about **1–2 hours after a meal**, in proportion to calorie intake.

Its functions include:

- **Slowing gut motility** (the "ileal brake"), prolonging digestion and satiety.

- **Signalling the brain** via the **vagus nerve** to suppress hunger.

- **Inhibiting ghrelin**, the hunger hormone.

Batterham et al. (2003) found that a single PYY infusion reduced buffet meal intake by 30%. Interestingly, **obese individuals had a weaker PYY response**, which may help explain persistent hunger despite higher food intake.

- ### Insulin – the post-absorption regulator

Insulin regulates satiety by acting on the brain — particularly the **hypothalamus** — to reduce hunger and signal fullness. While it is best known for its role in controlling blood glucose, insulin also functions as a **satiety hormone.**

How Insulin Regulates Satiety:

1. **Insulin is released after eating**, especially in response to carbohydrates.

2. It **crosses the blood-brain barrier** and acts on insulin receptors in the **hypothalamus**.

3. In the brain, insulin helps **suppress the activity of orexigenic neurons** (like NPY/AgRP) which stimulate appetite, and **activates anorexigenic neurons** (like POMC/CART) which suppress appetite.

4. This neural signaling **reduces appetite** and helps regulate **meal size and frequency**.

Chronically high insulin levels (as in insulin resistance or obesity) can blunt insulin's satiety signalling, leading to impaired appetite control. **Leptin and insulin** work in parallel as long-term regulators of body fat and energy balance.

- ### Leptin: The Metabolic Signal Regulator

Leptin is not a gut hormone. It is a hormone primarily produced by fat cells (adipocytes) that plays a key role in long-term energy balance. Unlike hormones like CCK or GLP-1, which act on a meal-to-meal basis, leptin helps regulate overall food intake and body weight over time.

Main roles:

- **Suppresses appetite:** Signals the hypothalamus to reduce hunger when fat stores are sufficient.

- **Regulates energy balance:** Helps the body maintain stable fat levels by influencing food intake and energy expenditure.

- **Acts as a satiety signal:** High leptin levels typically mean the body has enough energy, reducing the drive to eat.

However, in obesity, **leptin resistance** can develop. This means the brain no longer responds effectively to leptin's signals, causing persistent hunger despite high body fat levels—a major challenge in long-term weight regulation.

Another possible cause involves the ob gene, which encodes leptin—a hormone that signals the brain to curb appetite and boost energy use. When this gene is mutated and leptin is lacking, hunger regulation breaks down, leading to severe obesity. Though rare, it underscores leptin's vital role in energy balance.

These hormones work in a feedback system, adjusting food intake and energy use to maintain body weight. Alongside these key players, many other hormones and neuropeptides also shape appetite—some working short-term between meals, others managing long-term energy balance. While their roles are fascinating, diving deeper into them goes beyond the focus of this Book.

2.12   Can We Tap into Gut Hormones for Weight Loss?

If ghrelin sparks hunger and PYY signals fullness, could targeting these hormones be the key to weight loss? Research suggests it is not so simple.

Korner et al. (2003) found that blocking hunger hormones like ghrelin or AgRP has limited impact, as the body quickly activates backup systems. In contrast, disruptions in satiety pathways—such as MC4R, leptin, or POMC mutations—can lead to severe obesity, showing just how critical these appetite-suppressing systems are.

Interestingly, weight loss from **dieting** often **backfires** by increasing **ghrelin**, intensifying hunger and triggering rebound weight gain. Yet, gastric bypass surgery tells a different story: it lowers ghrelin while boosting PYY, helping people feel full and sustain weight loss more effectively.

We cannot easily override the body's natural weight-regulating mechanisms, and we are way behind in harnessing the power of PYY, ghrelin, related hormones or genes. However, knowing these we can work on how we could regulate this mechanism through our eating habits.

2.13   Food Intake Control Begins Before the First Bite

After my dissertation, emerged other studies that re-affirmed the importance of a preload or satiety starter. Brunstrom (2014) revealed something intriguing: our brain often decides how much we will eat before the first bite. We are guided initially by visual cues and expectations than actual calories. Foods that look and feel filling—like soups or potatoes—trigger stronger satiety signals than calorie-dense foods like chocolate or cheese, which often leave us unsatisfied despite their energy load.

Even more compelling is how distractions during meals—such as screens or multitasking—can dull memory encoding and reduce satiety, leading to increased food intake later. Conversely, simply reminding people of what they recently ate has been shown to reduce the amount consumed at a subsequent meal.

3   Preloads and their Effects on Satiety & Food Intake

Starting with this chapter, we embark on a journey through fascinating studies and insights that reveal how **food eaten before a main meal (preloads) can influence how much we eat afterward — and how well (or poorly) our bodies compensate for those extra calories**.

From this chapter onward to Chapter 8, you will find valuable insights and in-depth analysis. I have put great effort into making the content as clear and straightforward as possible because I know how important it is for you to understand the science behind these strategies. However, if you prefer a more concise overview, feel free to skip ahead to Chapter 9, where the key findings are summarised.

3.1   *Timing of the Preloads*

One of the earliest questions in preload research was timing—**how long before a meal** should a preload be consumed to **best influence** appetite and calorie intake?

Studies were done on timing using various types of preloads and comparing them:

- Carbohydrate and fat using yogurt
- Physical state using soup
- Fat and protein using omelette
- Liquid and solid foods

Research in this area began in the 1990s, with influential studies by Rolls et al. (1991), Spiegel et al. (1993, 1997), and Porrini et al. (1997) laying the groundwork. Later, Almiron-Roig et al. (2004) added new insights, particularly on how the physical form of preloads (solid vs. liquid) affects their impact. These studies provide a deeper understanding of how timing plays a role in regulating energy intake.

Coming up, Chart 1 offers a clear visual breakdown of how different types of preloads used in different studies, consumed at varying time intervals, influence overall energy intake.

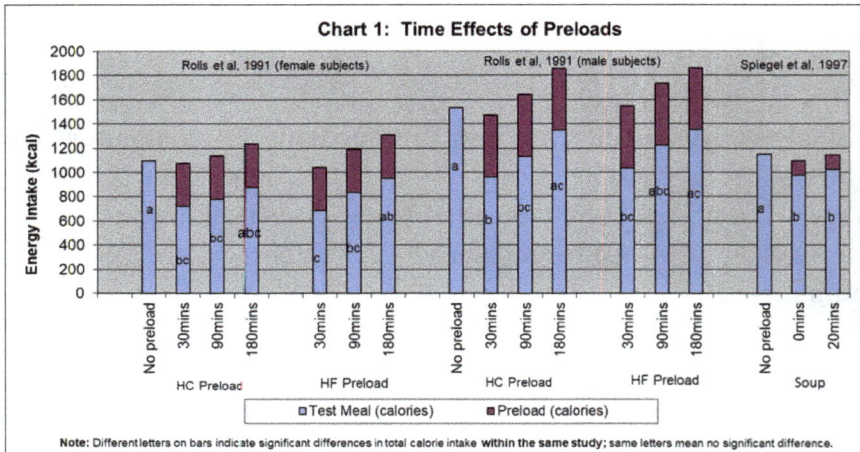

Chart 1: Time Effects of Preloads

Note: Different letters on bars indicate significant differences in total calorie intake within the same study; same letters mean no significant difference.

Here is what stands out with timing:

- **Closer Preloads = Stronger Effect** – When a preload is eaten right before or shortly before a meal, its impact is more noticeable. It not only reduces the energy intake of the meal itself but also lowers total energy intake (preload + meal).
- **Timing is Key, Even When Differences Are Subtle** – While not all variations in preload timing show statistically significant effects, the trend is clear: The closer the preload is to the main meal, the greater its ability to curb overall intake. Interestingly, when the preload is consumed too far in advance, total energy intake (test meal + preload) can sometimes surpass that of eating without a preload at all.

These findings underscore the potential of strategic preload timing as a simple yet powerful tool for managing food intake effectively.

Let us take a closer look at each study and break down the key findings in more detail. We will examine how different preloads, their composition, and timing influenced energy intake, satiety, and meal compensation.

3.2 Effects of High-Carb and High-Fat Yogurt at Different Timing

In a pioneering study, Rolls et al. (1991) investigated how preloading with high-fat (HF) or high-carb (HC) yogurt influenced hunger and food intake over time. Participants were given one of two preloads:

- High-Carb Yogurt (81% carbohydrates)
- High-Fat Yogurt (65% fat)

Each preload was consumed at different intervals before lunch:

- 30 minutes | 90 minutes | 180 minutes before eating.

Key Takeaways:

Best Results at 30 Minutes – When the preload was eaten 30 minutes before lunch, participants naturally compensated by eating less during the meal. Their bodies "remembered" the calories from the preload and adjusted accordingly.

The Longer the Wait, the Weaker the Effect – At 90 and 180 minutes, the body's ability to compensate became less accurate. By the 180-minute (3 hours) mark, those who had a preload ate just as much as or more than those who had not—suggesting the preload's impact had faded entirely.

Fat vs. Carbs? No Clear Winner – Interestingly, it did not matter whether the preload was high in fat or high in carbohydrates. Despite their very different digestion processes, both types of preloads had similar effects on hunger and meal intake.

The Big Lesson: If you want to use preloading to control hunger and reduce calorie intake, timing is crucial! According to this study, eating a preload around 30 minutes (or likely less) before a meal is most effective, while waiting too long weakens its impact.

3.3   What about a Soup at Different Timing?

Could a bowl of tomato soup actually slow digestion and help control appetite? Spiegel et al. (1993) put this to the test by giving nine female participants an egg sandwich breakfast under three different conditions:

- No Soup – Just the sandwich
- Soup Immediately Before – A 300g tomato soup right before the sandwich
- Soup 20 Minutes Before – Same soup, but with a delay

Key Findings

Soup Slows Digestion—But Only If Eaten Immediately Before: Researchers used radionuclide scintigraphy to track digestion and found that when soup was consumed right before the sandwich, it significantly slowed stomach emptying. However, when eaten 20 minutes earlier, this effect was greatly reduced.

Fullness Lasted for Nearly Two Hours: Both soup conditions led to **longer-lasting feeling of fullness** for up to 110 minutes after the meal compared to the no-soup condition. However, hunger ratings remained similar across all conditions. This suggests that while soup influenced feelings of fullness, it did not necessarily reduce hunger-driven eating cues.

What Does This Mean? The study suggests that the physical presence of food in the stomach plays a major role in satiety. When soup was present at the time of eating, it delayed stomach emptying and prolonged fullness. However, hunger signals are regulated by multiple mechanisms, and gastric (stomach-based) and post-gastric (digestive system-based) signals might counterbalance each other, leading to no significant change in overall hunger.

This study reinforces the idea that preloading with liquids could be a useful tool for appetite control—but **timing matters!**

3.4   *Best Time for Soup before a Meal?*

Building on their 1993 study, Spiegel et al. (1997) explored whether **timing of soup consumption** influenced food intake at a later meal. Participants were assigned to one of three conditions:

- **No Preload** – Ate lunch with no soup
- **Immediate Preload** – Had a **300g tomato soup** right before lunch
- **Delayed Preload** – Had the same soup **20 minutes before lunch**

Key Findings:

Soup Preloading Slowed Stomach Emptying

- **Immediate Preload:** Stomach emptying was slowest (**76.5 minutes lag time**).

- **Delayed Preload:** Shorter delay (**47.2 minutes lag time**).

- **No Preload:** Fastest digestion (**42.4 minutes lag time**).

- **More soup (125g) remained in the stomach** before they ate the sandwich in the **immediate preload condition** than in the delayed condition.

Reduced Meal Intake with Soup Preloading

- Participants who had soup **ate significantly less food at lunch** than those who did not.

- **Immediate preload resulted in slightly lower total calorie intake** than the **delayed preload and no preload.** But the total caloric difference between the two preloads timing was not significant.

Implications

This study suggests that preloading with **soup can effectively reduce food intake** at a subsequent meal, likely due to slower gastric emptying and prolonged satiety signals. Consuming soup immediately before a meal lowered energy intake – the suppressing effects lasted for about 20 minutes.

3.5   *High-Fat or High-Protein Omelettes at 0- and 120-min Interval*

Porrini et al. (1997) conducted a study examining how different preloads affected short-term energy intake. Participants consumed either a high-fat or high-protein omelette immediately before a lunch buffet. The results showed that **those who ate the high-protein omelette consumed fewer total calories (preload + lunch) compared to those who had the high-fat omelette**.

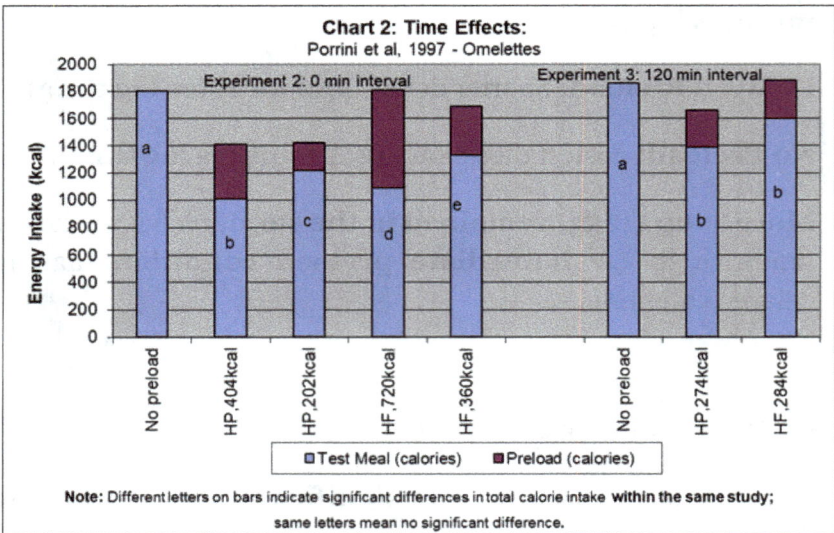

Chart 2: Time Effects:
Porrini et al, 1997 - Omelettes

Note: Different letters on bars indicate significant differences in total calorie intake **within the same study**; same letters mean no significant difference.

Chart 2 provides a summary of **total energy intake** based on the experiments conducted by Porrini et al. (1997). It visually represents how **preloading with high-fat (HF) and high-protein (HP) omelettes** at different time intervals before a meal influenced the participants' overall energy intake, highlighting key trends in their findings.

34

Interestingly, measured energy intake two hours after the preload and found that the **high-protein preload resulted in the lowest total energy intake**. However, the differences between the various conditions became less pronounced over time, suggesting that the impact of the preload on overall consumption diminished as time passed.

However, since the data came from two separate experiments, it is difficult to draw firm conclusions about the effect of timing. That said, comparing preloads consumed at 0 minutes versus 120 minutes, it appears that the body's ability to compensate for earlier calorie intake weakens as time passes.

3.6   *Sipping and Chewing at Different Timing*

Almiron-Roig et al. (2004) also found **compelling evidence for the impact of timing on food intake** while examining how the **physical state of a preload** influences subsequent eating behavior. Their study revealed that when participants consumed a preload just 20 minutes before a meal, their overall energy intake was significantly lower compared to those who had the preload 120 minutes prior. (This study is revisited in Chapter 7, where preload physical states are also examined, with results illustrated in Chart 5.) This finding reinforces the idea that timing plays a crucial role in how preloads affect hunger and calorie consumption—suggesting that the closer the preload is to the main meal, the stronger its impact on reducing overall intake.

3.7   *The Bottom Line*

These five studies collectively highlight a clear pattern: **the timing of a preload significantly impacts how well the body compensates for energy intake.** Rolls et al. (1991) found that within 30 minutes of consuming a high-carbohydrate (HC) or high-fat (HF) preload, energy compensation at the next meal was highly efficient. However, beyond this window, compensation for the additional preload energy dropped below 100%, and after three hours, the preload had little to no effect on energy intake. Interestingly, **different macronutrients influenced compensation over varying timeframes—Porrini (1997) observed that a high-**

protein preload still achieved full compensation at 120 minutes, whereas a high-fat preload never reached complete compensation.

Overall, these studies reinforce a key takeaway on timing: **the closer a preload is consumed to a main meal, the stronger its impact on reducing total energy intake.**

4 Effects of Volume in Preloads

Volume and energy density are often explored together in research, as it helps us understand better whether preloads can effectively reduce energy intake. In eight key studies, volume effects were examined under isoenergetic (same calorie) conditions, with energy intake from test meals carefully measured.

4.1 Volume of Preload Makes a Difference

Chart 3 brings together findings from three important studies on preloading:

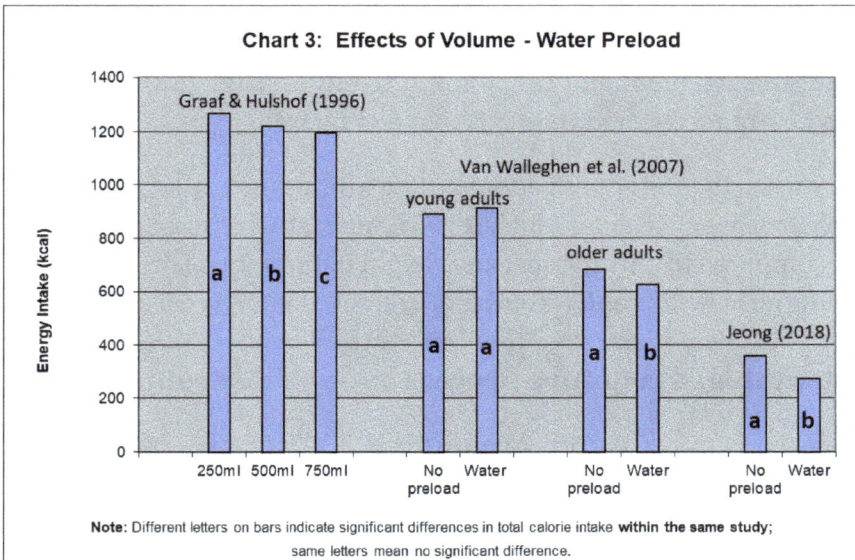

Chart 3: Effects of Volume - Water Preload

Note: Different letters on bars indicate significant differences in total calorie intake **within the same study**; same letters mean no significant difference.

Graaf and Hulshof (1996) explored how different preload volumes (250 mL, 500 mL, and 750 mL) and calorie levels (0, 300, and 600 kcal) influenced energy intake at a test meal. **Key takeaway:** As preload volume increased, food intake at the meal significantly dropped. In short — the more you drink before eating, the less you eat afterward.

Van Walleghen et al. (2007) found something similar. They tested pre-meal water (375 mL for women, 500 mL for men) in younger (21–35) and older adults (60–80). After drinking water, older adults ate significantly less at lunch, while younger adults showed little change.

Jeong (2018) reaffirmed that **volume matters**. In young, non-obese adults, drinking 300 mL of water immediately before a meal reduced calorie intake — although it did not notably increase fullness.

The difference between Jeong's and Van Walleghen's findings on younger adults might lie in **timing**: in Van Walleghen's study, water was consumed **30 minutes before** the meal, giving the body time to register fullness signals. In Jeong's, it was taken **immediately before** eating. A subtle but important detail: when it comes to preloading, timing counts.

A randomised controlled trial by Parretti et al. (2015) strengthened the real-world case for water preloading. Eighty-four adults with obesity were advised on weight management and randomised to either drink 500 mL of water 30 minutes before meals or simply imagine feeling full.

Over 12 weeks, the water preloaders lost an average of **2.4 kg** — twice as much as the control group. Remarkably, **27%** of them shed at least 5% of their body weight, compared to only **5%** lost any weight in the control group. Consistency mattered: those who drank water before all three main meals saw the greatest results. This also illustrates that an **actual water preload is more important than a cognitive process and self-restrain**.

The message is clear: **water preloading is a simple, affordable, and powerful tool for weight management** — no extreme diets required. And if plain water alone can deliver such results, even greater success may lie ahead when more effective preload strategies are used — a topic we will explore in the coming chapters.

4.2 *Volume and Calories Working Together*

In six of the seven studies (see Chart 4), consuming a preload with calories before a meal led to a decrease in subsequent energy intake, with the effect becoming stronger as preload volume increased. But what happened to the total calorie intake (test meal + preload)?

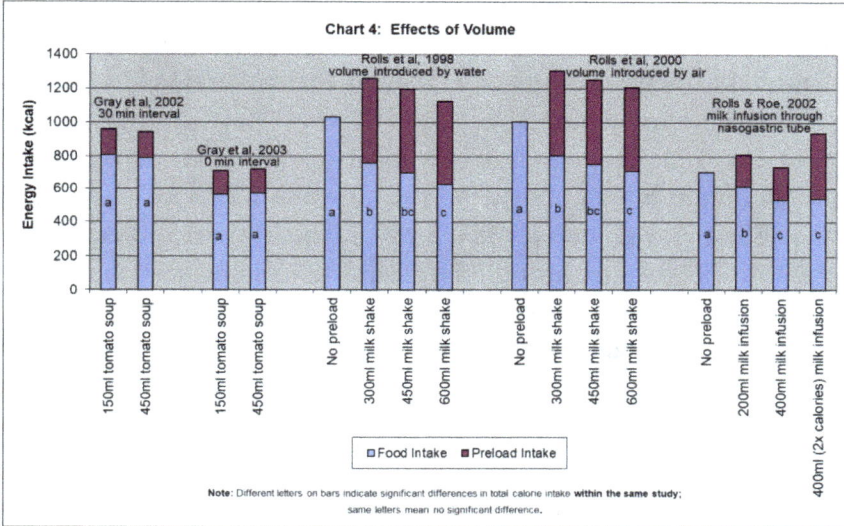

Chart 4: Effects of Volume

Significant Findings in Two Studies Rolls et al. (2000) & Rolls & Roe (2002) illustrated in Chart 4—found a statistically significant reduction in food intake in the test meal when comparing a no-preload condition to a preload condition - the higher the volume, the lesser the intake at test meal. However, it is worth noting that **total energy intake**, the combined calories from the preload and the meal **exceed those of the no-preload condition** – a trade-off we will address in upcoming chapters.

An Exception: Westerterp & Verwegen (1999) Unlike the above studies, Westerterp & Verwegen (1999) found no significant difference between the no-preload condition and a 340ml zero-calorie water preload for both male and female participants (Chart 12). However, a caloric milkshake preload of the same volume did significantly reduce subsequent food intake.

Why the Difference? While Rolls et al. (2000) observed significant effects with a 300ml preload, the null response in Westerterp & Verwegen (1999) suggests that **volume alone is not the only determining factor—caloric content also plays a key role** in influencing satiety and subsequent intake

4.3   *Impact of Liquid Preload is Short-lived*

In most of these studies, total short-term energy intake—including both the preload and the meal—was higher than in the no-preload condition. The standout exception was Spiegel et al. (1997), where participants compensated for 95% of the total preload and test meal energy when it was consumed immediately before lunch, and fully (100%) when taken 20 minutes earlier. This hints at just how **fleeting** the effects of **liquid preloads** can be—likely due to their rapid passage through the stomach. Gamma scan data confirmed this: although participants consumed a 300 g soup preload, only 125 g remained in the stomach at mealtime. Remarkably, **a mere 20-minute shift in timing altered compensation by 5%,** underscoring how quickly liquids lose their appetite-suppressing edge.

4.4   *Gender Differences in Response to Food Volume and Intake*

Rolls et al. (2000) found that increasing preload volume only **significantly reduced** food intake when raised from **300 ml to 600 ml**. Similarly, Rolls & Roe (2002) observed a **decrease in intake** when increasing volume from **200 ml to 400 ml** (both at 200 kcal). However, doubling the calories to **400 kcal** at the same **400 ml volume** did not affect intake—suggesting that **volume** matters more than **calories** alone. The volume effect was more pronounced with larger increases: **200 ml for women** (Rolls & Roe, 2002) and **300 ml for men** (Rolls et al., 2000).

In contrast, Gray et al. (2002, 2003) found that boosting preload volume from **150 ml to 450 ml** (at 150 kcal) had **no impact on intake in men**, but raising the energy to **450 kcal** did. Interestingly, under intragastric conditions, Rolls & Roe (2002) did observe volume effects.

The mixed results might be due to **gender differences** or differences in **cognitive and sensory responses**. Rolls studied women, while Gray focused on men—suggesting that **women may be more sensitive to volume changes**, while **men respond more to energy content**.

5 Effects of Energy in Preloads

Eight studies explored how volume and energy content affect food intake, with several also examining the roles of perception and social context. While the results are mixed, distinct patterns — and intriguing contradictions — begin to emerge.

5.1 Volume vs Energy

To isolate the body's physiological response, Rolls & Roe (2002) used intragastric infusions of milk-based preloads, bypassing taste and visual cues. They found that volume influenced intake, but energy density did not. (Chart 5)

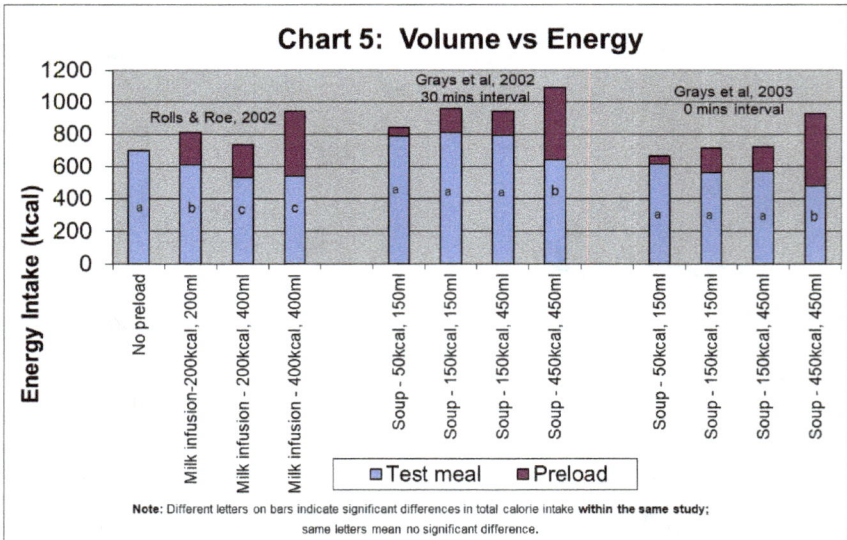

Chart 5: Volume vs Energy

Note: Different letters on bars indicate significant differences in total calorie intake within the same study; same letters mean no significant difference.

In contrast, Gray et al. (2002, 2003), using soup preloads consumed either 30 minutes or immediately before a meal, found the opposite: energy density influenced intake, but volume did not. One likely reason for the discrepancy? Gender differences, as observed earlier in Section 4.4. Rolls studied women;

Gray studied men — **reinforcing the idea that women may respond more to volume, and men more to calories**. (Chart 5)

5.2 *Effects of Energy Content and Other Influences*

Other studies examined how volume and energy density influence food intake, while also considering the roles of perception, social setting and macronutrient composition. These diverse methodologies provide a well-rounded understanding of how volume, energy density, perception and macronutrient shape eating behaviours. (Chart 6)

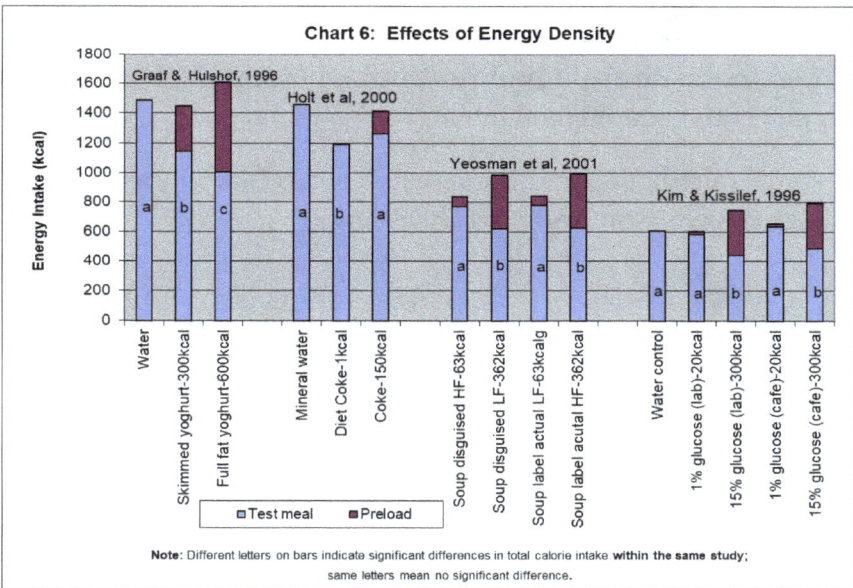

Chart 6: Effects of Energy Density

Note: Different letters on bars indicate significant differences in total calorie intake **within the same study**; same letters mean no significant difference.

- **Energy density:** Graaf & Hulshoff (1996) compared the effects of **skimmed vs. full-fat yogurt** on subsequent food intake. **Increased energy density reduced subsequent food intake** but overall energy intake (test meal + preload) is not compensated with the full-fat yoghurt.

- **Real-world beverage choices:** Holt et al. (2000) examined how calorie differences in widely consumed beverages—**Diet Coke versus**

43

regular Coke—affected later intake of potato crisps and a buffet meal. Surprisingly, **diet coke with almost no calorie had effect** on subsequent food intake as does than original coke. **Sweetness overshadows energy content.**

- **Perception vs reality:** Yeomans et al. (2001) explored the role of perception by disguising the energy content of preloads (labeled as high-fat or low-fat) and comparing them to accurately labeled controls. The **disguised labels did not significantly affect intake**; the actual energy levels did.

- **Social context and sugar concentration:** Kim & Kissileff (1996) investigated whether the social setting (eating in a lab versus a cafeteria) influenced intake after consuming 500ml of 1% or 15% glucose preloads. While **social context had no impact**, higher glucose concentration significantly reduced food intake.

These studies also highlight those actual preloads **has higher effects than cognitive perception and social settings**.

Macronutrients with Different Energy Content

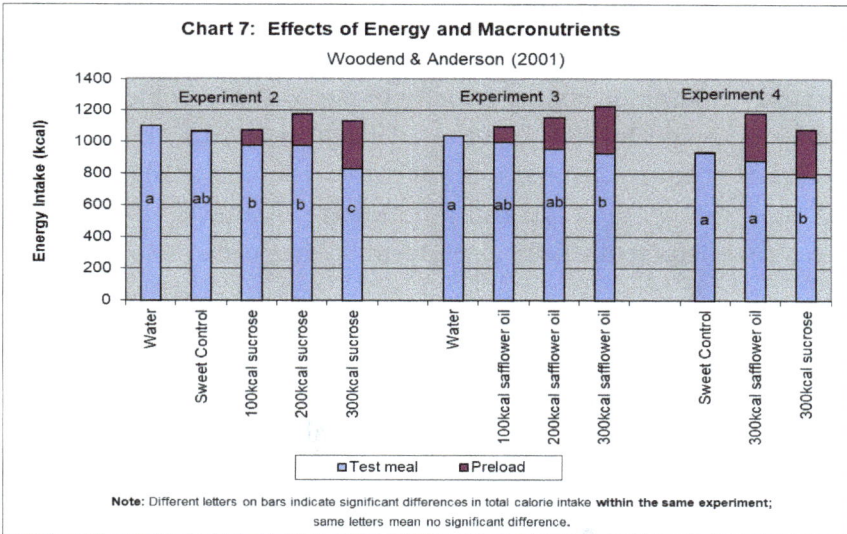

Chart 7: Effects of Energy and Macronutrients
Woodend & Anderson (2001)

- Woodend & Anderson (2001) ran four experiments to test how sucrose and safflower oil, at varying energy densities, influenced food intake. They found that higher energy density reduced subsequent intake — with sucrose proving more effective than oil. However, this **reduced intake did not fully offset the extra calories from the preload.** The effects of macronutrient will be examined further in the next chapter.

5.3   *Is there an Energy Threshold?*

Charts 5–7 show that most studies — except for Holt et al. (2000) — found that higher preload energy content reduced subsequent food intake. However, the effect was not always statistically significant, and at higher energy densities, compensation was often incomplete.

Holt et al. stood out: **Diet Coke, despite being almost zero-calorie, influenced intake much like regular Coke**, hinting that **sweetness,**

not calories, shaped response — a finding echoed by Anderson & Woodend (2003).

Gray et al. (2002, 2003) confirmed that **total energy content of the preload**, not volume or energy density alone, was the key driver for **male test subjects**. At low levels (50–150 kcal at 150-450 mL), energy density had no impact. But at equivalent densities at higher volumes at higher energy level (450 mL at 450kcal), the total energy content did affect intake. Simply put, **volume alone was not enough especially for men**.

Gender plays a role. Rolls & Roe (2002) suggested that **men respond more to energy increases** than women, pointing to possible biological differences in satiety signalling. Across studies, a clear pattern emerges: a ~300 kcal increase appears to be the tipping point for reliably reducing food intake — for male participants.

These findings suggest an energy threshold — a point where the body recognises the preload and adjusts intake — along with a likely gender difference: women respond more to volume, men to calories.

5.4   *Striking the Right Energy Balance in Preloads*

As preload energy increases, compensation rarely keeps pace — meaning total energy intake (preload + meal) often ends up higher than if no preload was consumed. In Graaf & Hulshof (1996), compensation was near complete, likely because the preload was small (20% of the test meal at 300 kcal, but not at 600 kcal), and consumed just 15 minutes prior (Chart 6). This effect held across preload volumes of 250 ml, 500 ml and 750 ml.

The studies reviewed so far suggest that there is a minimum effective preload energy. For women, **300 g of tomato soup** (Spiegel et al., 1997) was effective at about **10% of the test meal's energy**. For men, an approximate **9% preload** using a **sucrose solution** (Woodend & Anderson, 2001) was noted.

To guide practice, a 9–10% preload energy threshold may be sufficient to ensure full compensation. **Beyond 20%, total calorie intake may rise above that of no preload instead of fall.**

A systematic review and meta-analysis by Rouhani et al. (2017), done after the completion of my dissertation, strongly supports these patterns. Reviewing 39 studies, they found that **low energy-dense (LED) preloads — typically rich in water or fibre — consistently reduced total energy intake** compared to high energy-dense (HED) ones. However, they also warned of delayed compensation: LED preloads may lead to increased intake later in the day, especially at dinner or during evening snacking. This underscores the importance of strategic timing—**targeting your largest or latest meal of the day is likely the most effective approach**.

6 How Macronutrients Influence Satiety Over Time

Macronutrients—carbohydrates, proteins, and fats—are processed differently by the body, each following distinct metabolic pathways. As a result, they may influence appetite and energy intake in different ways, depending on when their effects are measured.

Thirteen studies have investigated how specific macronutrients influence subsequent food consumption, offering valuable insights into which nutrients are most effective at curbing appetite—and how long their effects last.

To capture these differences, the impact of various **macronutrient preloads** has been analysed across **multiple time intervals**: immediately (0 minutes), and at 30, 60, 90, 120, 180 minutes, and beyond. This time-based breakdown allows for a clearer **comparison of how each nutrient affects hunger and intake over time**.

6.1 Effects of Protein

Among all macronutrients, **protein consistently shows the strongest satiety effect**. Even small amounts of protein or fat before a meal can help moderate blood glucose by **slowing gastric emptying**, which reduces post-meal spikes (Nesti et al., 2019).

These effects appear even **more pronounced** in individuals with **type 2 diabetes (T2D)**, making protein preloads especially useful for improving glycaemic control. Additionally, protein-rich foods are typically **less energy-dense than fats**, making them an efficient choice for preloading.

Protein's role in appetite regulation has been examined in **seven key studies**, which show that it often outperforms carbohydrates and fats in controlling hunger and reducing subsequent intake.

The charts below illustrate how protein preloads affect food intake over time:

- **Immediate effects (0 min):** Chart 8

- **Short-term effects (20-30 min):** Charts 12

- **Moderate-term effects (90 min):** Chart 9

- **Longer-term effects (120 min):** Chart 9

- **Extended effects (300 min):** Chart 10

- **Effects when used as a snack preload:** Chart 11

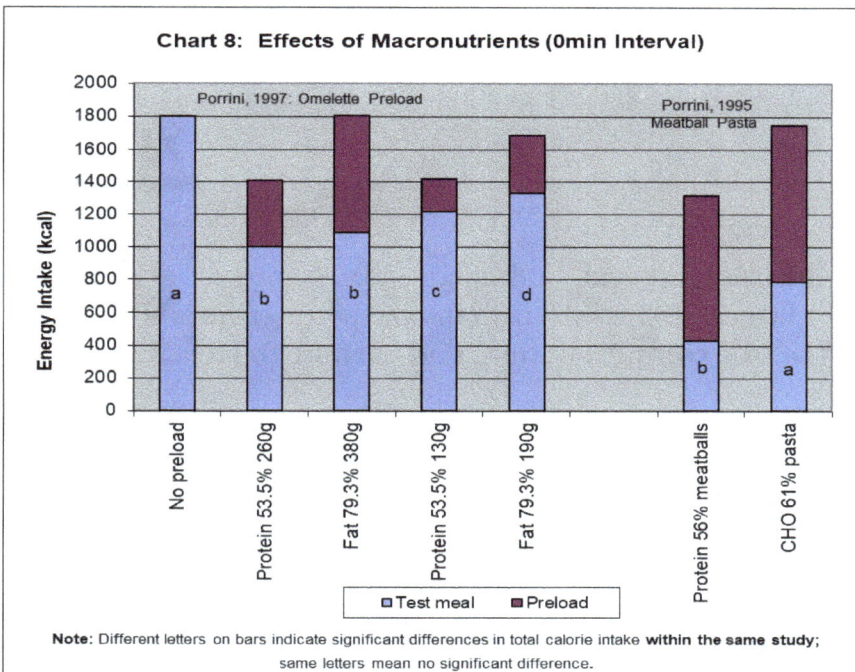

Chart 8: Effects of Macronutrients (0min Interval)

At 0 minutes: Porrini et al. (1995, 1997) used omelette and meatball pasta as preload. They found that **protein significantly reduced subsequent energy intake** compared to both fat and carbohydrates. **Total calorie intake was well compensated** and significantly below that of the preload (see Chart 8).

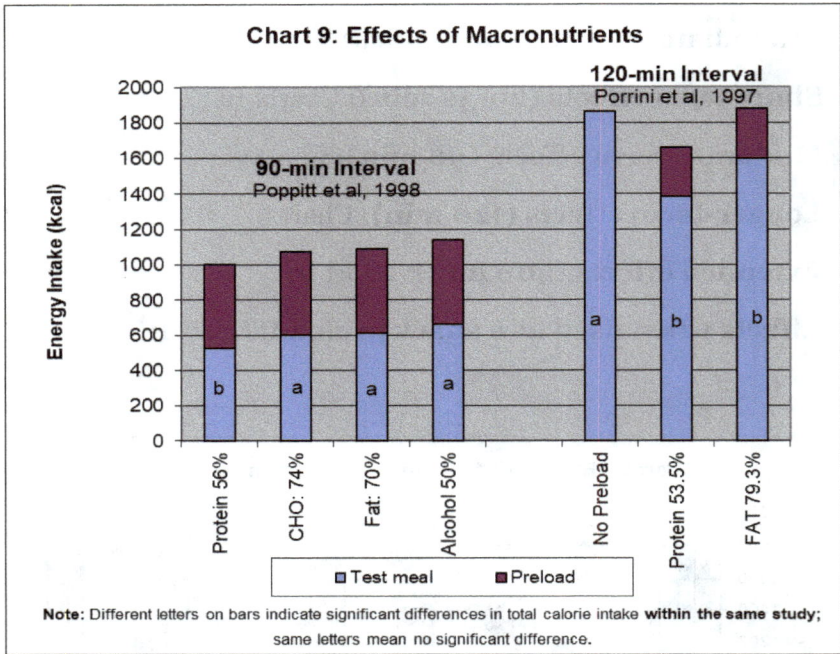

Chart 9: Effects of Macronutrients

Note: Different letters on bars indicate significant differences in total calorie intake **within the same study**; same letters mean no significant difference.

At 90-minute interval: A similar effect of protein was observed **90 minutes later**, with Poppitt et al. (1998) reporting a **notable suppression of total intake compared to fat and carbohydrate** preloads (Chart 9).

At 120 minutes, protein still significantly suppressed intake compared to no preload (Porrini et al., 1997; Chart 9). However, its advantage over high-fat preloads diminished, suggesting protein's appetite-suppressing edge may fade with time. **Crucially, though, total energy intake was more than compensated for—leading to a net reduction in calories.**

These findings suggest that **protein's impact on appetite suppression is strongest within the first two hours. But this effect may taper off over longer durations compared to fat.**

6.1.1 When Studies Show No Effect — Why is that Still Insightful?

Interestingly, some studies—like those by Raben, Johnstone, and Westerterp—found no clear macronutrient winner for appetite control. Why?

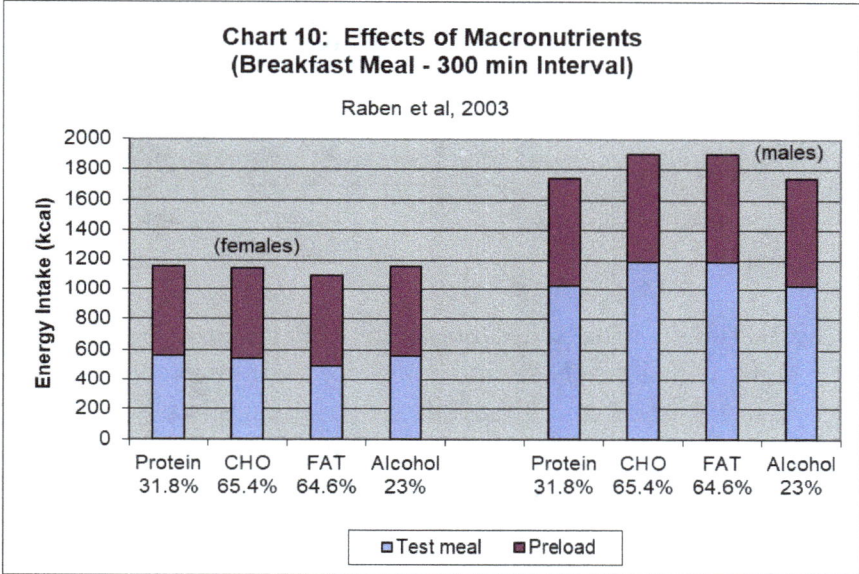

Chart 10: Effects of Macronutrients (Breakfast Meal - 300 min Interval)

Raben et al, 2003

Extended 5-hour interval: The lack of significant findings in Raben et al. (2003) could be attributed to the extended 5-hour interval, which far exceeds the 120-minute threshold observed in Poppitt et al. (1998). Additionally, the protein content in Raben et al.'s study was relatively low at 31.8%, meaning its effects may have been diluted by the presence of other macronutrients. (Chart 10)

Chart 11: Effects of Macronutrients (Snacks)

Johnstone et al, 2000

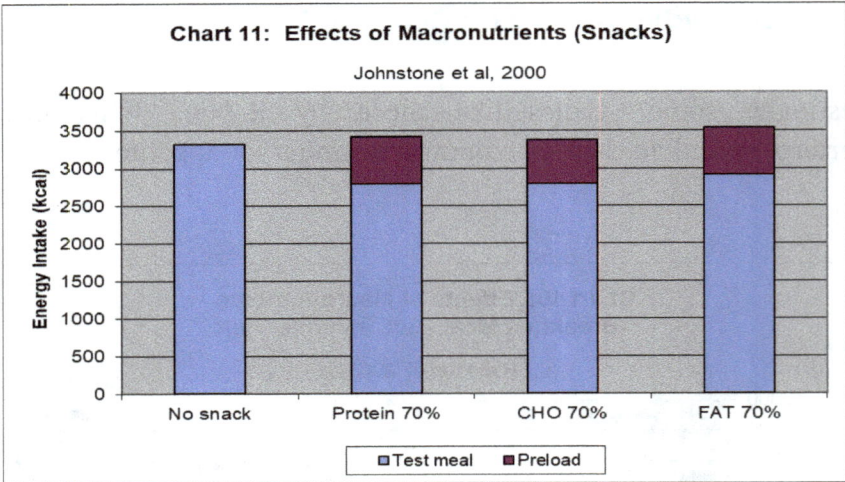

Snacking Between Meals: In Johnstone et al. (2000), snacks were given 1.5 to 2.5 hours before meals—long enough for their effects to wear off. This likely reflects inter-meal snacking rather than preloading. The total calorie intakes for all four macronutrients exceed the no-snack scenario. The key takeaway? **Snacks** are **forgotten by mealtime**, **adding calories** without reducing intake—an easy way for weight to creep up. (Chart 11)

Fluids vs solids: An intriguing contrast emerges when comparing Westerterp & Verwegen (1999) with the studies by Porrini et al. (1995, 1997). Westerterp & Verwegen found no significant difference between protein and carbohydrates and fat. (Chart 12).

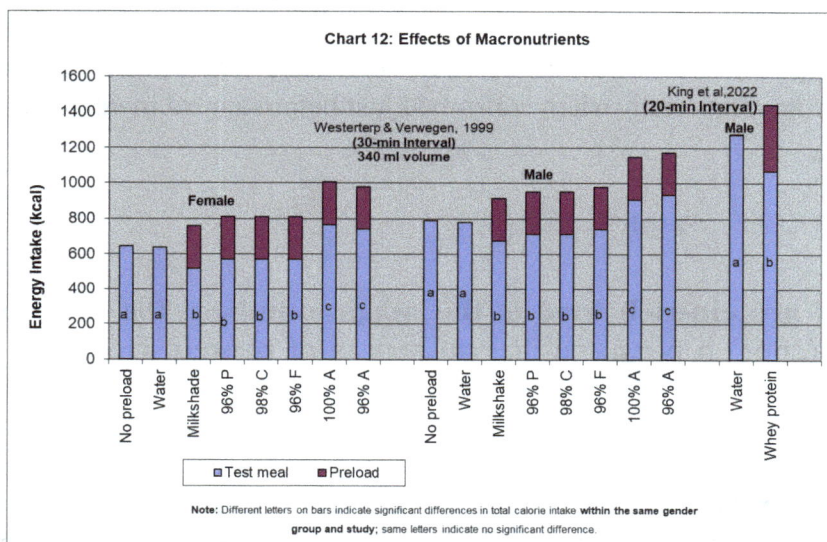

Chart 12: Effects of Macronutrients

The key difference lies in the form of the protein preload. Westerterp & Verwegen (1999) used a **protein-enriched fruit juice,** made by adding Protein 88 (Sandoz Nutrition) to a fruit-flavoured drink, whereas Porrini et al. (1997) used **low-fat ham** and Porrini et al. (1995) used **meatballs** to enhance protein content. Meanwhile, Poppitt et al.'s study (Chart 9) involved **fish and potato pie** alongside a gin and tonic, though the additional protein content was unspecified.

Following my dissertation, **King et al. (2022)** found that a **20 g whey protein preload (~90 kcal) in water** taken **20 minutes before a pasta meal** reduced energy intake by **16–18% (207 kcal)** in both healthy-weight and overweight men. There was **no compensatory eating or change in activity** over 48 hours, but **total energy intake within the test meal +**

preload was not fully compensated. This aligns with **Westerterp & Verwegen (1999)**, where protein in fluid form also showed limited compensation.

This contrast raises an intriguing question: **Does the form of protein matter?** Solid, whole-food sources like meat may deliver greater satiety than liquid protein drinks, thanks to their denser structure and slower digestion.

Overall, **protein is most effective at reducing food intake** compared to carbs or fats, especially when consumed just before a meal in **solid form**.

6.1.2 Other notable findings

50g of protein-rich food is the magic number: The Anderson and Moore (2004) paper noted that **50 grams of protein-rich food** is the tipping point for real satiety. Below that, the effects are hit-or-miss — especially when fats and carbs get thrown into the mix. But once you cross the 50-gram mark, studies consistently show **greater fullness, reduced hunger, and lower food intake**. If you want to truly harness the power of protein to curb your appetite, **50 grams is where the magic starts**. (Anderson and Moore 2004). This is an important number to note when planning a pre-meal.

No synergistic effect of protein and fat: Oesch et al. (2005) tested whether combining an oral protein preload with intraduodenal (ID) fat perfusion would enhance satiety more than either alone. In this double-blind crossover study, 20 healthy men completed four conditions. Protein preload alone cut intake by **19%**, fat perfusion alone by **11%** (not significant). Combining protein and fat cut intake by 27%, but because the combination carried double the calories, total energy intake still exceeded that of the controls. **Combining protein and fat does not amplify satiety beyond their separate effects**.

Reduced post-meal blood glucose: In the Smith et al. (2021) study, a **15 g whey protein preload (100 kcal)** taken 10 minutes before a fixed pasta meal **reduced post-meal blood glucose by 13–18%** in both lean and centrally obese. The test meal was identical across conditions, isolating the effect of the preload. The benefit was linked to **increased GLP-1 (Glucagon-like Peptide-1)** and **slower gastric emptying**, though the GLP-1 response was weaker in obese test subjects. Despite the extra calories, **appetite and total intake remained unchanged**.

6.2   *Effects of Carbohydrates and Fat*

Compared to carbohydrates and fats, protein preloads consistently prove more effective at reducing calorie intake.

The power of carbohydrates to satisfy hunger is a mixed bag — **complex carbs** like whole grains keep you fuller longer, while **simple sugars** offer far less staying power. **Fat**, though rich in energy and able to slow digestion, is surprisingly poor at curbing appetite. It is easy to overeat, quietly adding extra calories. While fats are important for **absorbing fat-soluble vitamins** and providing **essential fatty acids**, foods high in fat are best enjoyed **in mindful amounts**.

Among the eight preload studies that directly compared carbohydrate and fat preloads, nearly all found no significant differences between the two—except for the intriguing findings of Woodend & Anderson (2001), where a subtle but noteworthy variation emerged. (Studies include those examined earlier as well as Rolls et al. 1991 &1994 and Cecil et al, 1998)

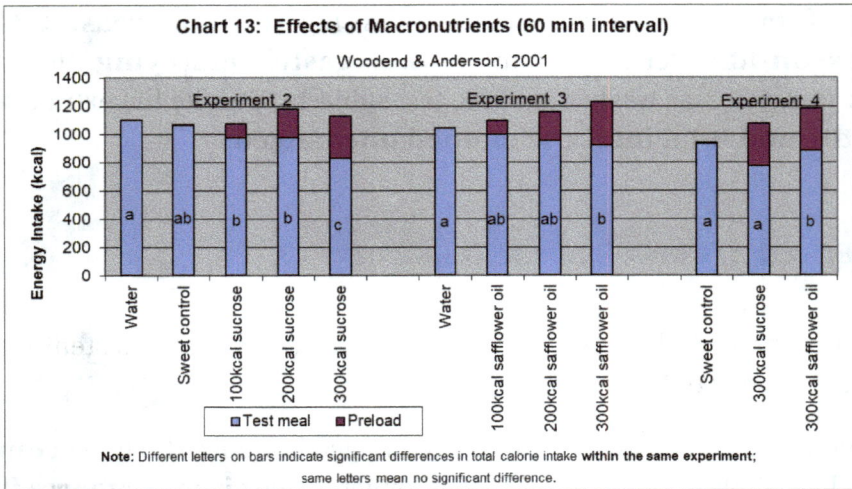

Chart 13: Effects of Macronutrients (60 min interval)
Woodend & Anderson, 2001

Note: Different letters on bars indicate significant differences in total calorie intake **within the same experiment**; same letters mean no significant difference.

The study by Woodend and Anderson (2001) is striking for its simplicity — using pure macronutrient preloads: **100% fat** (safflower oil) and **100% carbohydrate** (sucrose solution). They found only an **8% difference in calorie compensation**, hinting that the body responds slightly differently when processing these nutrients alone. Yet despite these shifts, **total calorie intake still rose** compared to no preload at all, showing that simply manipulating macronutrients is not enough to drive weight loss. (Chart 13)

Interestingly, **carbohydrates had a stronger short-term appetite-suppressing effect than fat, but this advantage quickly fades once other macronutrients are mixed into a meal.**

Carbs vs fat in weight loss: In an 8-week study after my dissertation, Johnston et al. (2013) discovered that **preloading with a carbohydrate-rich grain bar** (140 calories) before dinner led to a significant **weight loss of 1.3 kg**, compared to just **0.2 kg** in the group consuming a **fat-rich peanut bar preload** (166 calories). This striking difference highlights how easily the **body compensates for lower-calorie** carbs, but struggles to self-regulate after higher-fat preloads.

6.3   Effects of Fibre

Fibre pulls double duty: it slows digestion, fills you up, and adds barely any calories. Fruits, vegetables, and whole grains which are fibre-rich foods not only pack fibre but also deliver a bonus of vitamins and antioxidants. Soluble fibre, in particular, shines by slowing gastric emptying and stretching out the feeling of fullness — but its impact on cutting calories later is modest (Andersen and Moore, 2004).

While **fibre beats simple carbs and fat** when it comes to satiety, it does not pack the same punch as protein. Andersen and Moore (2004) pointed out that **fibre works best when teamed up with other satiety boosters**, like high-protein foods and low energy-dense meals. Fibre helps, but for real appetite control, **pairing it with protein is a winning strategy**.

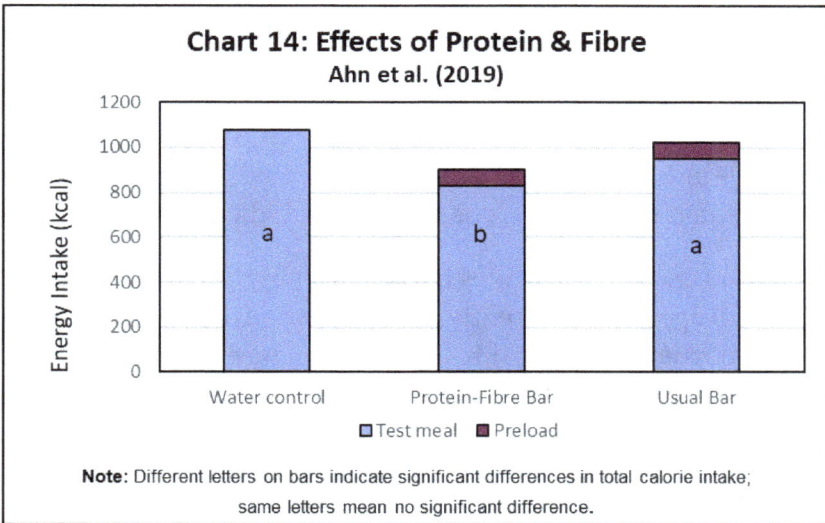

Chart 14: Effects of Protein & Fibre
Ahn et al. (2019)

Note: Different letters on bars indicate significant differences in total calorie intake; same letters mean no significant difference.

Ahn et al. (2019) tested whether a protein-enriched, fibre-fortified bar (PFB) could curb appetite better than an isocaloric usual bar (UB) or water. Both bars provided 73 kcal, but the PFB packed in 10.7 g of protein and 12.7 g of fibre, while the UB had hardly any. After eating freely at a test meal, participants who had the PFB consumed significantly fewer calories than after water (904 vs. 1,075 kcal). The PFB also boosted fullness, enhanced GLP-1 secretion, and improved post-meal blood sugar control. (Chart 14)

Even a small protein and fibre preload made a real difference without adding unwanted calories. Reductions in food intake tracked more closely with rises in PYY than GLP-1, pointing to a key driver of satiety. These results suggest that a modest, well-designed preload could be a simple yet powerful tool for appetite and weight management.

6.4   *Effects of Sugars and Sweeteners on Satiety and Intake*

Anderson and Woodend (2003) highlighted two key points in their review:

- **Sweetness itself can influence appetite** — low-calorie sweeteners reduced hunger and intake, even without calories. This suggests **taste alone can modulate satiety**, as seen in Holt et al. (2000), where diet cola surprisingly suppressed food intake.

- **Fructose may be more effective than glucose** in reducing intake—but only under certain conditions. Its advantage vanished when eaten with other carbs, like cereal, indicating context matters.

Different sugars and carbohydrates trigger varying glycemic responses, which may influence appetite differently. **Anderson and Woodend (2003)** concluded that **sugars and high-GI carbs** reduce short-term food intake more effectively than low-GI carbs or fats (but not necessary the total energy intake of meal + preload). However, this effect likely involves more than just blood glucose changes—**satiety peptides and digestive timing** also play important roles.

Van de Ven et al. (1994) showed that **fructose combined with high fibre** significantly reduced intake at 30 minutes, while low-fibre versions did not, suggesting a **synergistic effect**.

Overall, the impact of sugars on satiety depends on sugar type, amount, nutrient pairing, and digestive duration.

Lee et al. (2021) reviewed 35 studies and found that **low-/no-calorie sweetener (LNCS) preloads** reduced energy intake compared to **unsweetened ones**. However, when matched for sweetness, LNCS preloads led to slightly higher subsequent intake than **caloric sweeteners**, but total daily intake was still lower—indicating only **partial compensation** for the energy in caloric versions. (Holt et al., 2000 supports this, as shown in Chart 6.)

Not all low- or no-calorie sweeteners (LNCS) reduce energy intake; some have even been linked to increased appetite, alongside ongoing safety concerns in certain cases. I remain cautious and choose not to include them in my preload strategy—at least until the evidence becomes more conclusive.

6.5   Effects of Alcohol on Subsequent Food Intake

Alcohol's influence on appetite has been explored in five preload studies. The Caton et al. (2003) and Yeomans & Philip (2000) studies specifically compare lager at different alcohol concentration.

In Caton et al (2003), participants who consumed an 8% alcohol lager showed a 9% increase in food intake compared to a no-alcohol lager, and a 16% increase compared to a 2% alcohol lager. This suggests that **higher concentrations of alcohol may stimulate appetite**, even when the accompanying energy and volume are greater. (Chart 15). Notably, the appetite-stimulating effect was **not observed** with the lower 2% alcohol lager. (Note: Alcohol content is reported by weight, not by percentage of energy.)

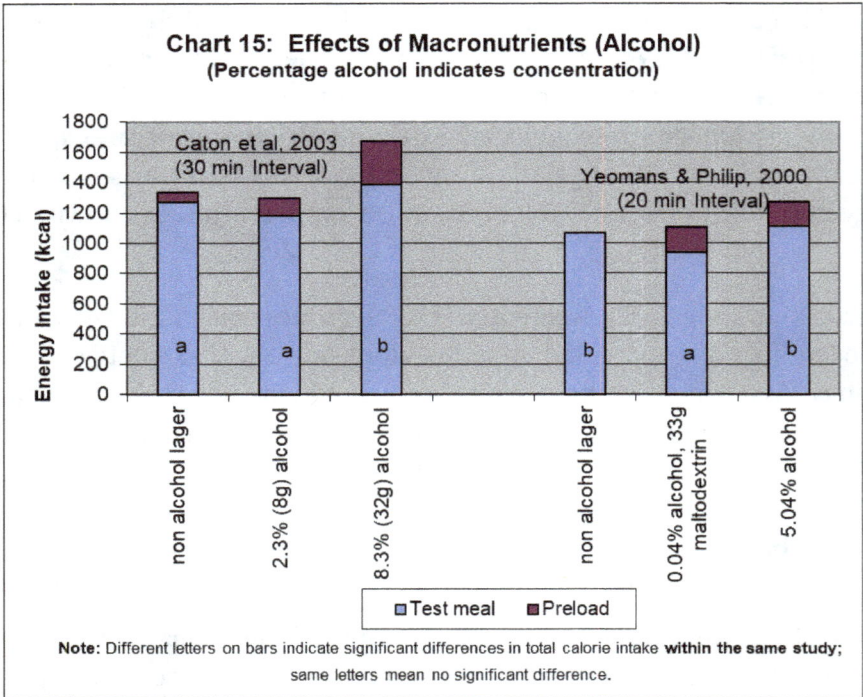

Chart 15: Effects of Macronutrients (Alcohol)
(Percentage alcohol indicates concentration)

Caton et al, 2003 (30 min Interval)

Yeomans & Philip, 2000 (20 min Interval)

Note: Different letters on bars indicate significant differences in total calorie intake **within the same study**; same letters mean no significant difference.

In **Yeomans & Phillips (2000)**, a 5% alcohol lager led to a higher food intake than water, although the difference was not statistically significant. However, when compared to a 0.04% alcohol lager matched in calories using maltodextrin, the increase was significant, suggesting that the **presence of alcohol itself**, not just its energy content, **influences appetite**. (Chart 15).

Westerterp & Verwegen (1999) found that alcohol preloads resulted in **higher food intake** compared to other macronutrients (see Charts 10). The food intake was also higher than the no preload and water preload condition although not significantly different.

Similarly, **Poppitt et al. (1998)** observed that alcohol led to the **highest energy intake** relative to protein, fat, and carbohydrate preloads, although again, the difference was not significant.

Only **Raben et al. (2003)** found **no notable effect** of alcohol compared to the other macronutrients. However, this study used a **5-hour interval** between breakfast and lunch, which may have allowed the appetite-stimulating effects of alcohol to wear off.

Taken together, these findings suggest that **alcohol's caloric value is poorly regulated by the body**, with higher concentrations (above 5%) possibly **stimulating rather than suppressing** appetite. This contrasts with other macronutrients, which tend to reduce food intake in the short term.

7 Effects of Physical State

There have been claims that the body's ability to detect and regulate ingested energy is less precise for liquid beverages than for solid foods. However, the evidence remains inconclusive, as variations in study outcomes may be influenced by factors such as subject characteristics, preload volume, and the time interval between the preload and the test meal.

Four key studies—Almiron-Roig (2004), Rolls et al. (1999), Himaya & Sylvestre (1998), and Hulshof & De Graaf (1993)—specifically examined how the physical state of preloads affects subsequent energy intake. A summary of their findings is presented with energy intake trends visually mapped in Chart 16.

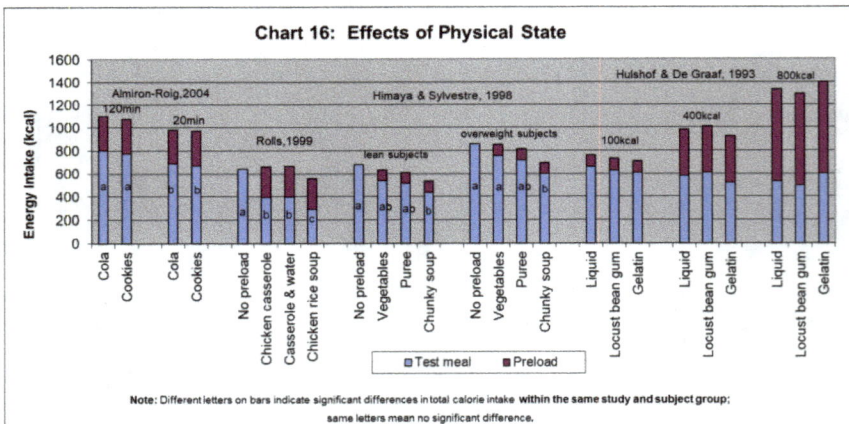

Chart 16: Effects of Physical State

Although no significant difference was found between solid and liquid preloads in total calorie intake across these studies, an interesting trend emerged. It turns out that solid preloads are generally more satisfying than liquid ones. However, two studies—Rolls et al. (1999) and Himaya & Sylvestre (1998)—unearthed some intriguing findings that challenged this idea.

7.1 An Intriguing Finding – Chunky Soups

Rolls et al. (1999) discovered that **chicken rice soup had a significantly greater effect on reducing food intake than a chicken casserole paired with a glass of water**, even though both had the same ingredients, energy content, and volume. Similarly, Himaya & Sylvestre found that **chunky soup had a stronger effect than puree vegetables**, even though both were made of the same ingredients, energy, and weight. This effect was seen across both lean and overweight groups. (Chart 16).

The chicken rice soup preload at 270 kcal saw a compensation rates of 87% of total energy intake for females. The chunky tomato soup preload of 95 kcal saw a 85% compensation rate for overweight males. (These compensation rates are calculated based on total energy intake for each of the preload scenario divided by the energy intake for the no preload.)

These were the lowest compensation percentages (most effective) observed across all the studies comparing physical states, highlighting a unique finding—**mixing solid food with liquid led to a greater reduction in food intake** than consuming either solid food or liquid alone, or even a solid food paired with a drink of equal volume.

7.2 Solid Fruits vs Liquid Alternatives

Following my dissertation, Flood-Obbagy et al. (2009) explored how 4 different forms of apple — whole segments, applesauce, and apple juice (with or without fibre) — influenced satiety and energy intake at a meal. (Chart 17) Despite matching preloads for calories, weight, energy density, and ingestion time, whole apples stood out: they led to the greatest reduction in total lunch intake and left participants feeling significantly fuller compared to applesauce or juice. Applesauce had a modest effect, while both types of juice did little to curb appetite or lower intake. Notably, adding fibre to apple juice offered no real advantage over regular juice.

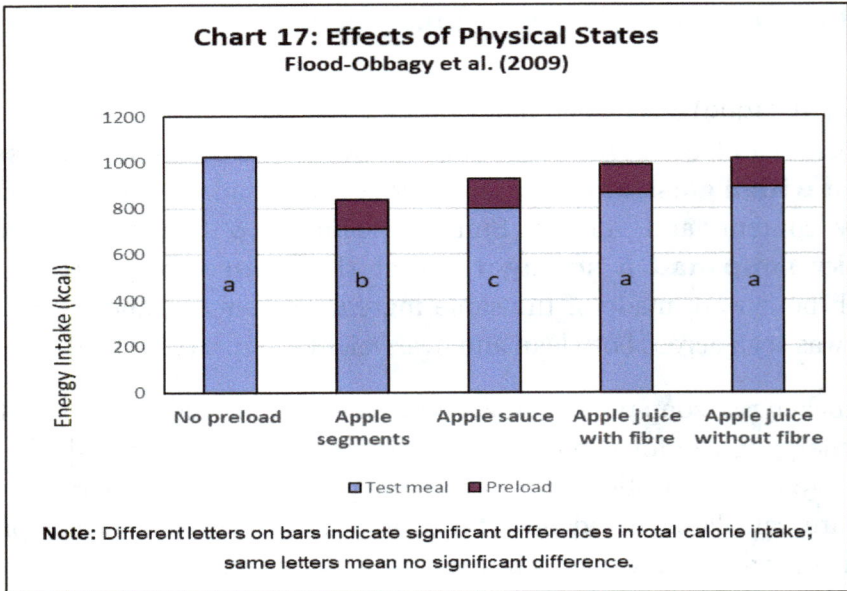

Chart 17: Effects of Physical States
Flood-Obbagy et al. (2009)

Note: Different letters on bars indicate significant differences in total calorie intake; same letters mean no significant difference.

The study makes one thing clear: **the physical form of food matters**. Solid foods like **whole fruits are far more effective** at promoting fullness and managing calorie intake **than pureed or liquid versions** — even when nutrients are matched. **Chewing and food structure**, not just fibre content, **amplify satiety**. These findings reinforce the value of whole fruits over juices or purees as a simple, effective tool for appetite control.

Solid foods outperform fluids in both making you feel full during a meal (satiation) and keeping you full after the meal (satiety) (Bellisle et al., 2012).

The Stribiţcaia et al. (2020) systematic review and meta-analysis explored how food texture — from form (solid, semi-solid, liquid) to viscosity and complexity — shapes appetite and energy intake. Across 29 studies, **solid foods consistently reduced hunger more than liquids, and thicker, high-viscosity foods boosted fullness better than thinner ones.** While solids only slightly lowered later food intake, added texture — like seeds or aeration — showed early promise in enhancing satiety. Gut hormones (CCK, GLP-1, PYY, ghrelin) were less reliably influenced with liquid foods.

8   Behavioural Differences between Lean & Obese Groups

One of the intriguing aspects explored in this dissertation is the difference in behavior between obese or overweight individuals and those of normal weight, especially in response to pre-meals or preloads.

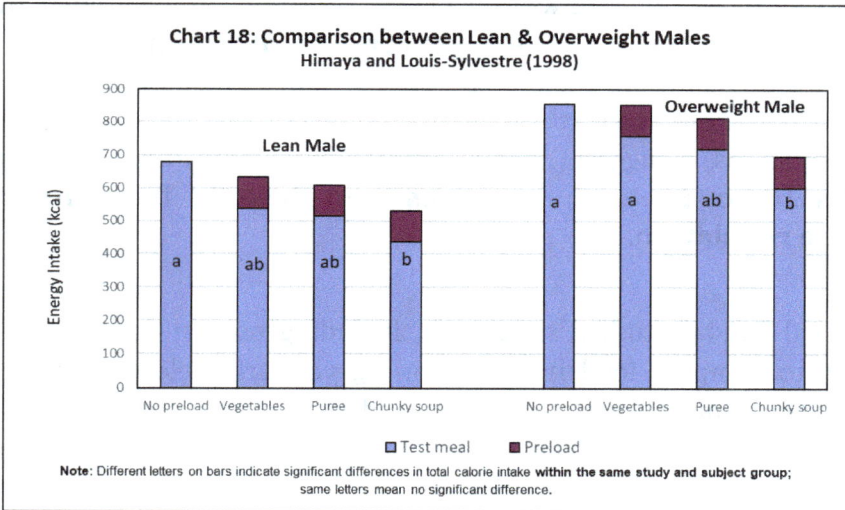

Chart 18: Comparison between Lean & Overweight Males
Himaya and Louis-Sylvestre (1998)

Note: Different letters on bars indicate significant differences in total calorie intake **within the same study and subject group**; same letters mean no significant difference.

Rolls & Roe (2002) investigated whether lean and obese women would respond differently to preloads when traditional visual and oral cues were bypassed, with food being infused directly into the stomach. Interestingly, they found no significant difference in the way the two groups responded. Both groups suppressed subsequent food intake equally, suggesting that when sensory cues are removed, the **behavioural response to food intake may be similar, regardless of body weight**.

Rolls & Roe's finding strongly supports the concept of using **preloads** as a practical strategy to reduce energy intake. Since the study shows that **volume-based satiety effects** work similarly for both lean and obese individuals, it reinforces the idea that **high-volume, low-calorie pre-meals** can be an effective tool for appetite control regardless of body weight.

Westerterp and Verwegen (1999) focused on the effects of different macronutrient preloads, such as fats, carbohydrates, and proteins, on energy intake. While they observed some differences between male and female subjects, there was no significant difference between overweight and normal-weight participants when it came to the energy intake.

In the Himaya and Louis-Sylvestre (1998) study, both lean and overweight participants responded similarly to preloads of different physical states. Notably, although the **overweight group** consumed more at lunch overall, they **demonstrated a higher percentage of compensation** when comparing preload to no-preload conditions—indicating they **reduced their intake more relative to their baseline**. (Chart 18). This finding is highly encouraging, as it suggests that **overweight individuals can respond effectively to preload strategies and benefit from improved appetite regulation.**

Rolls et al. (1994) studied six groups, including normal-weight and obese women, to compare food intake following yoghurt preloads with varying carbohydrate and fat content. They found that, overall, obese participants consumed more than their normal-weight counterparts.

While the normal-weight group fully compensated for preload energy, the obese group showed only partial compensation—except for a 262-kcal medium-high carbohydrate yogurt, which was fully compensated. This suggests that although the **obese group** did adjust intake, they were **less effective at compensating for high-fat and high-carb preloads**. This highlights the lower satiating power of these macronutrients for the overweight. (Chart 19)

Chart 19: Comparison between Lean and Obese Females

Rolls et al, 1994

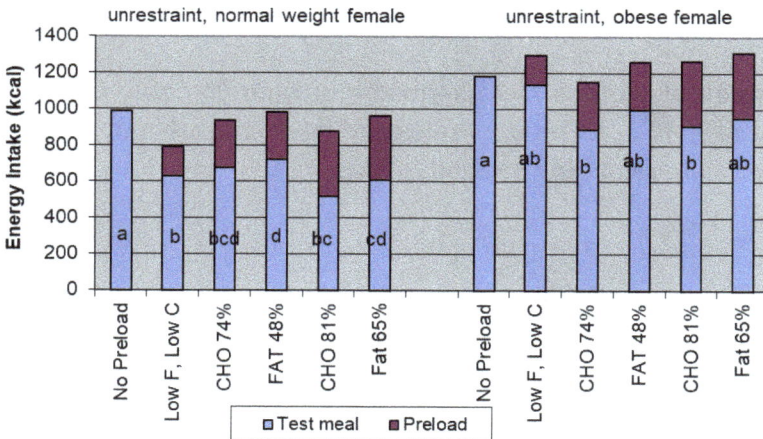

Note: Different letters on bars indicate significant differences in total calorie intake **within the same study and subject group**; same letters mean no significant difference.

In summary, while overweight and obese individuals do respond to preloads similarly to those of normal weight, their ability to compensate for the additional energy appears less efficient. These studies indicate that the **obese may have a reduced sensitivity to the satiating effects** of **fats and carbohydrates**—which can contribute to greater overall intake. This has important implications for individuals with obesity — they need to pay particular attention to reducing high-fat and high-carbohydrate foods, as these are easy to overeat.

However, the evidence consistently points to **chunky soup as a powerful tool for appetite control**, even among those with obesity, offering a practical and effective strategy to help manage hunger and reduce calorie intake.

9 Pulling It All Together

The interplay of various factors—macronutrients, energy content, volume, and physical state—creates a complex and fascinating dynamic when it comes to the effects of preloading on food intake.

1. Timing Makes all the Difference: The timing of a preload shapes how it influences appetite. **The strongest effects occur when eaten immediately before a meal**—what researchers call "zero interval." Protein preloads, for example, can suppress intake even after 120 minutes (Porrini et al., 1997), while carbs and fats lose their edge by 30 minutes (Rolls et al., 1991). Spiegel et al. (1997) showed the impact fades fast for liquids—pureed soup preloads worked best only when taken less than 20 minutes before eating.

Why? The stomach reacts quickly and triggers satiety signals even before full digestion begins. The small intestine contributes, but slower. This fast response helps regulate intake before food is absorbed.

Interestingly, **the idea of eating frequent small meals is refute by this observation**. Without strict calorie control, people tend not to compensate for extra intake—especially from snacks spaced out too long from meals. So, in reality, this approach is not natural and only works if people can exercise enough self-control to avoid overeating.

2. Volume Helps, but Nutrients Matter More: Drinking water alone may reduce food intake but **nutrient-rich** preloads **generate stronger satiety** responses. Read et al. (1994) found stomach stretch is not enough; satiety hormones need nutrients to kick in. For noticeable effects, men need ~300 mL of liquid, women ~200 ml.

3. Enough Energy, But Not Too Much: Spiegel et al. (1997) found that the body can only compensate for preload calories up to about 10% of a meal's energy.

Rolls et al. (1991), however, saw better compensation (30%+). One likely reason for the stronger compensation is the buffet-style lunch, which offered more low-calorie options like fruits and vegetables, allowing participants to unconsciously adjust their intake. In contrast, Spiegel et al. used a fixed egg sandwich meal, likely higher in energy density, leaving less room for natural adjustment.

Compensation tends to fail when preload energy exceeds ~300 kcal. This makes low energy density foods more forgiving, as the body handles them better. These findings highlight the advantage of low energy density foods, which the body is better equipped to adjust for. This aligns with broader research suggesting that our physiology is more adept at preventing starvation than curbing overeating.

4. Protein Takes the Lead in Hunger Control. Among calorie-containing macronutrients, protein is the most effective at curbing appetite, followed by fibre, carbohydrates, and fat. Alcohol, by contrast, tends to stimulate appetite, particularly at higher concentrations.

Protein's satiety effects are rapid, likely triggered in the stomach before absorption, and can last up to two hours. In contrast, carbohydrates and fats tend to lose their impact within about an hour.

According to Anderson and Moore (2004), approximately **50 g (1.76 oz) of protein-rich food is the tipping point for a meaningful satiety response**, particularly when consumed just before a meal.

Marmonier et al. (1999) found that protein-rich snacks delayed the next meal by an average of 60 minutes, compared to 34 minutes for carbohydrates and 25 minutes for fats. However, total energy intake still increased with snacking, suggesting that snacking may not support weight control in individuals prone to weight gain.

5. Fibre - The Unsurprising Hero of Satiety: When it comes to activating fullness, fibre proudly takes the silver medal—just behind protein. It is a powerhouse addition to your meals, not only because it helps keep you satisfied but also because fibre-rich foods like vegetables and fruits are packed with vitamins and antioxidants. Plus, non-starchy veggies give you all that goodness without piling on the calories.

6. The Power of Nutrient Combinations: Pure fat or sugar does not suppress appetite like mixed meals do. A high-protein liquid (96% protein) was less effective than a mixed meal with protein, carbs, and fat—like meat stew. The **body responds best to complex nutrient combinations**, not isolated macros.

7. Solid Foods in Soup is the Winner: Soups with solid ingredients—like chicken rice or chunky tomato—consistently reduce intake more than solid, liquid or puree alone (Rolls et al., 1999; Himaya & Sylvestre, 1998). One possible explanation is that **a chunky soup involves the combination of chewing, volume and the fast dispersion of nutrients when it reaches the stomach.** Each of these contributes to achieving the food suppression effect.

8. Overweight Individuals Respond to Preload: Overweight individuals tend to eat more at test meals (Pearcey & Castro, 2002), but still respond to preloads—albeit less efficiently than those of normal weight (Rolls et al., 1994). Notably, chunky soups remain highly effective, even in this group, offering a promising strategy for appetite management (Himaya & Sylvestre,1998).

To empower this group to take control of their eating habits, a hearty chunky soup as a starter or appetizer offers an exciting opportunity—unlocking innovative strategies for managing excessive food consumption.

10 Designing the Pre-Meal Satiety Starter (or Appetizer)

After diving deep into the research on preloads and uncovering how all the key factors come into play, let us now unlock the secret to crafting a powerful pre-meal satiety starter or appetizer, the practical application of a preload, that tames your appetite, enhances satiety, and drives a substantial reduction in overall calorie intake.

If we want a satiety starter we will actually stick to—something we reach for before diving into our main meals—it needs to tick a few key boxes:

- It must fit easily into our daily routine,

- Offer enough variety to keep things interesting,

- Be quick and simple to prepare,

- And most importantly, it must be genuinely healthy.

Because if it is not practical, enjoyable, and good for us, it will not stand the test of time.

Building on the key findings summarised in the previous chapter, here are my top picks for pre-meal satiety starters that are not only effective but also delicious and satisfying:

- **Chunky soups** — hearty and comforting, that meet the volume, macronutrient and energy sweet spot to help curb appetite naturally.

- **Fresh salads** — crisp and refreshing, especially when paired with a drizzle of light dressing or a spoonful of low-fat yogurt.

- **Whole fruits** — juicy, vibrant, and full of natural fibre, these are a flavourful way to ease into your main meal.

Each of these options feels like real food—wholesome, enjoyable, and designed to keep you feeling full without overdoing it.

11 Pre-Meal Satiety Starter Recipes

Hindsight is perfect. When I began this research, I had no idea what truly boosted satiety, curbed cravings, or prevented overeating – the path forward was uncertain. But now, with the full picture in focus, the answer feels almost obvious.

With the satiety starter, you now have another powerful tool in your toolbox to help curb overeating, support weight loss, and maintain the weight you have worked hard to lose. By harnessing the science of fullness and meal timing, this simple strategy can make a lasting difference—helping you stay in control, eat more mindfully, and build sustainable habits for long-term success.

11.1 Tasty Soups to Satiety

A hearty, chunky soup is not just comforting—it is a proven way to kick-start your meal and naturally reduce calorie intake. Research shows that when eaten just before your main course, a soup that is **low in energy density** and **at least 300 ml in volume** can significantly boost satiety. This volume is key for effectiveness across both men and women.

To keep things simple, I use "meat" to refer to animal-based proteins such as poultry, beef, lamb, venison, seafood, and eggs. "Plant-based proteins" include wholesome options like lentils, tofu, beans, and peas.

Whether you are a meat-eater or plant-focused, **adding protein and fibre** to your soup does more than just curb hunger—it **amplifies nutrition**. For soups with meat, aim for **about 50g (1.76 oz)** of protein and **1 cup of vegetables** to trigger that satisfying fullness.

If you prefer plant-based proteins, check **Appendix D and E** for exact quantities of lentils, legumes, tofu, and other alternatives that match the calorie value of 50g of meat (82 kcal).

These recipes strike the ideal balance: **filling but not heavy**, **flavourful yet calorie-conscious**. Their warmth, texture, and ease of preparation make them simple to enjoy and easy to stick with.

My approach is straightforward: **eat well, without wasting time**. If that resonates with you, you are in the right place. These recipes are practical, quick to prepare, and health-focused—without compromising on taste.

Because let us face it—**healthy eating only works if the food tastes good.** And these meals are more than fuel; they are experiences that nourish both body and spirit.

At the heart of every recipe are **non-starchy vegetables**—vibrant, nutrient-rich, and low in calories. When paired with quality protein, they create meals that support your wellness goals while delivering real satisfaction. **Good food should taste as good as it makes you feel.**

To get you started, I have created **8 soup starter recipes** inspired by global flavours—including **4 plant-based options** (see Chapter 12). These soups are **chunky, not blended**, to maximise satiety and keep you feeling fuller for longer. While these recipes were developed with the help of **artificial intelligence**, I have given precise instructions, and personally checked and verified every detail to ensure they are both accurate and effective.

They are **customisable and easy to adapt**—you can swap meats, change up the veggies, and tailor the flavours to suit your pantry and preferences. Since protein-rich foods add more calories, portion sizes are carefully managed in the higher-energy soups.

Each recipe serves **one**, but scaling up for a family is easy—just multiply the quantities.

The satiety starter recipes in Chapter 12 include:

Satiety Starters – Chunky Soups	
Animal-based protein	**Plant-based Protein**
1. Chunky chicken & vegetable soup 2. Chunky beef & vegetable soup 3. Hearty curry fish & veggie soup 4. Boxing-day turkey veggie soup	1. Hearty lentil & eggplant soup 2. Spinach & white bean soup 3. Miso tofu seaweed soup 4. Chunky tomato & pea soup

11.2 Customising to Your Preference

Everyone's needs and preferences are different—what works for one person might not work for another. That is the beauty of it: you get to **explore, experiment, and discover what keeps you full, satisfied, and on track**, bearing in mind the goal is to **keep meals low in energy density**.

You can also adapt your satiety starter soups using a simple, flexible formula: **50g of meat + 1 cup of firm vegetables** (like carrots or turnips) per serving. If using leafy greens, go with **2 cups uncooked** and tightly packed as they shrink significantly once cooked. *(1 cup = 240–250 ml)*

If you prefer **plant-based proteins**, the same principle applies. Simply substitute the meat with ingredients like **lentils, tofu, beans, or peas**—using the energy-equivalent amounts listed in **Appendices D and E**. These guides help you match the **82 kcal** found in 50g of meat, so you stay on track without guessing.

To help you make informed choices, **Appendices B and C** list the caloric values of common ingredients— to help you create soups that are both satisfying and low in calories.

Everyone responds differently to these starters. If you find you need something more filling to curb your intake at the main meal, the lower energy-dense approach is to add water or broth, and vegetables. Try adding **half to one** cup of vegetables and enough water or broth to bring it to your desired volume. This simple combination increases fibre, nutrients, and volume, helping you feel fuller with minimal added calories.

I usually enjoy my soups clear and chunky. But if you prefer a thicker, creamier texture, you can absolutely adjust—**just bear in mind that thickening adds calories**, which may not always be offset. A **½ tsp of cornstarch slurry** adds about **10 kcal**, while **1 tbsp of cream** adds around **30 kcal** per serving.

Every bowl is an opportunity to eat well—**flavour-packed, nourishing, and light in energy**.

11.3 Salads as a Smart and Vibrant Satiety Starter Choice

When you want a break from soup, a fresh salad is a great satiety starter option. Western-style meals often begin with a salad for good reason—it sets the tone and helps curb overindulgence later.

Salads are easy to prepare and pre-pack options are readily available from the supermarkets. But watch the dressings—many are calorie-heavy. Try making your own: blend **1 cup each** of extra virgin olive oil, fruit or apple sauce, and apple cider vinegar, plus 1 tablespoon (tbsp) Dijon mustard. It keeps well in the fridge and is a tasty way to use up fresh seasonal fruits. For a quicker option, a small tub of low-fat yogurt can make a quick, fuss-free dressing. As there are easy, convenient options available, I would not provide any salad recipes in this Book.

11.4 Whole Fruits

Whole fruits can also serve as an effective and convenient satiety starter option. Their natural fibre content, high water volume, and low energy density help promote fullness without adding excessive calories. Among the best choices are apples, oranges, pears, and berries—fruits that require chewing, offer volume, and have a low glycaemic load. These not only slow eating but also engage the senses, increasing the feeling of satiety.

Avoid fruit juices or purees as satiety starter, since their liquid form and rapid digestion result in weaker appetite suppression. When choosing whole fruits, opt for those with skin (like apples or pears) and structure over softer or higher-sugar varieties like bananas or grapes. Used wisely, whole fruits make a portable, refreshing, and nutrient-rich pre-meal strategy.

11.5 *Take Charge when Eating Out*

Dining out can feel like a challenge when it comes to staying on track—menus are often fixed, loaded with tasty but not always healthy choices. But you are not powerless! Here is how to take charge:

Start with a **glass of water, a low-calorie, non-alcoholic beverage or a chunky soup** to kickstart your fullness. Next, move on to the **salad**—filling up on fibre before tackling the rest. Then focus on the **protein** dishes, saving **starches or fried items for last**. This simple order can naturally help you eat less without feeling deprived – by then, you need less of the energy-dense foods. Do not order dessert until you have finished your main course—you might find you no longer want it. If you feel full before finishing, do not force it; pack the rest for later or leave it behind. And if you consistently have leftovers, consider adjusting your order next time.

If your local spot serves mountains of **rice or fries**, confidently ask for a **half portion of these**—small changes like this can make a big difference. Plus, if more diners start requesting healthier portions, eateries might just catch on and adjust their serving sizes, making dining out a bit healthier for everyone.

12 Satiety Starter Recipes – Chunky Soups

These soups may be light, but they are purposefully designed to help curb your appetite before your main meal—without adding extra calories. Looking for heartier options? Check the next chapter for how to create main course soups that can stand alone as a light meal.

12.1 *Chunky Chicken & Vegetable Soup – Satiety Starter*

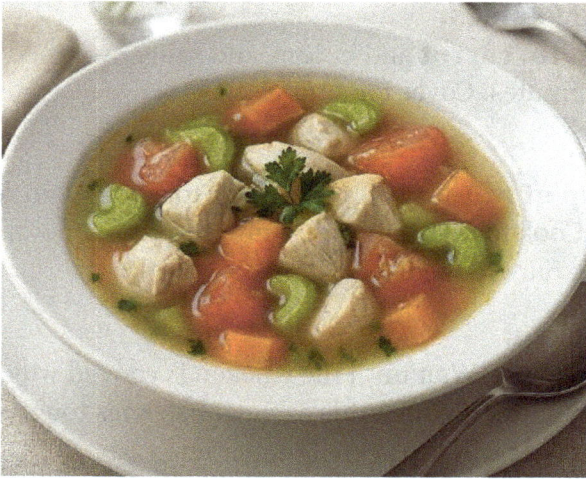

Serves: 1 | Prep + Cook Time: ~15–20 minutes | Calories: ~130–140 kcal

Ingredients:

- **50g (1.8 oz) chicken breast**, sliced or diced (about 1/3 small chicken breast)
- **1 garlic clove**
- **½ cup carrot**, peeled and sliced
- **½ cup celery**, chopped
- **½ medium tomato**, diced
- **¼ small onion**, chopped

- ¼ **tsp olive oil** or canola oil (optional)
- **1 cup water** (or low-sodium chicken broth)
- Salt and pepper to taste
- Optional: a clove of garlic, chopped parsley, or a few drops of lemon juice

Instructions:

1. **Sauté the aromatics:**
   In a small pot, add ¼ **tsp oil** (or a splash of water) over medium-high heat. Add onion and garlic, sauté until soften.

2. **Sauté vegetables:**
   Add **tomato, carrot** and **celery** and sauté over medium-high heat for 2–3 minutes. Cover for 5 minutes.

3. **Simmer:**
   Add **1 cup of water** (or broth). Bring to a boil, then reduce to a simmer. Cook for 8–10 minutes until the vegetables are tender and chicken is fully cooked.

4. **Add chicken:**
   Stir in **chicken**. Wait until the chicken is cooked which should be under 2 minutes. (Watch this as meat becomes tough when over-cooked and we want to keep it tender and tasty.)

5. **Season and serve:**
   Add **salt and pepper to taste**. Garnish with herbs or a dash of lemon if desired. Serve hot.

Estimated Nutrition (per serving):

Protein: ~11–12g | Fat: ~7–8g (with oil) | Carbohydrates: ~6–7g | Fiber: ~2g

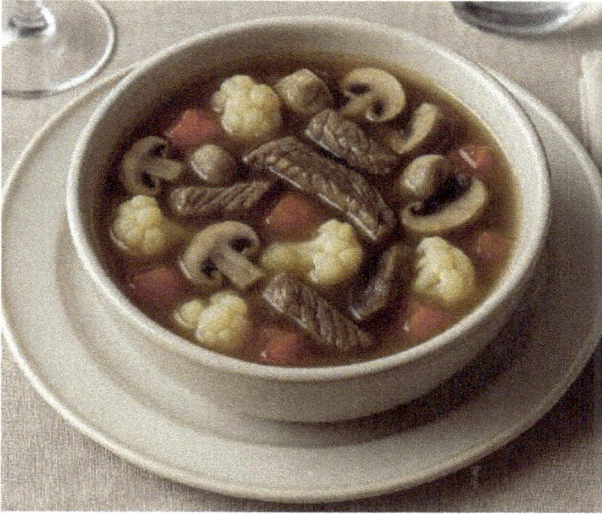

Serves: 1 | Prep + Cook Time: ~15–20 minutes | Calories: ~130–140 kcal

Ingredients:

- **50g (1.8 oz) thinly sliced beef** (e.g. flank steak, strips of sirloin, or shaved beef)
- **¼ tsp oil** *(optional)*
- **1 garlic clove**
- **¼ small onion**, chopped
- **½ medium tomato**, diced
- **2/3 cup cauliflower florets**, chopped small
- **1/3 cup mushrooms**, sliced (any variety; e.g. button or shiitake)
- *(Vegetables total ~1 cup when combined)*
- **1 cup water** (or low-sodium beef broth)
- **1/2 tsp oil** *(optional)*
- **Salt and pepper to taste**
- Optional: minced garlic, chopped parsley, thyme, or a squeeze of lemon

Instructions:

1. **Sauté aromatics:**
   In a small pot, heat ¼ **tsp oil** or a splash of water. Add onion and garlic and sauté until soften.

2. **Sauté vegetables:**
   Add **cauliflower, mushrooms, and tomato**. Sauté for 2–3 minutes until lightly softened.

3. **Simmer:**
   Add **1 cup water or broth**, season with **salt and pepper**, and bring to a gentle boil and simmer until the vegetables are soft.

4. **Add beef.**
   Stir in the **beef slices**. Cook until the beef is no longer pink, which should be under 2 minutes. (Avoid over-cooking the beef as it would become tough.)

5. **Finish and serve:**
   Turn off the heat. Taste and adjust seasoning. Garnish with fresh herbs or a touch of lemon juice if desired.

Estimated Nutrition (per serving):

Protein: ~13–14g | Fat: ~6–7g | Carbohydrates: ~5g | Fiber: ~1.5g

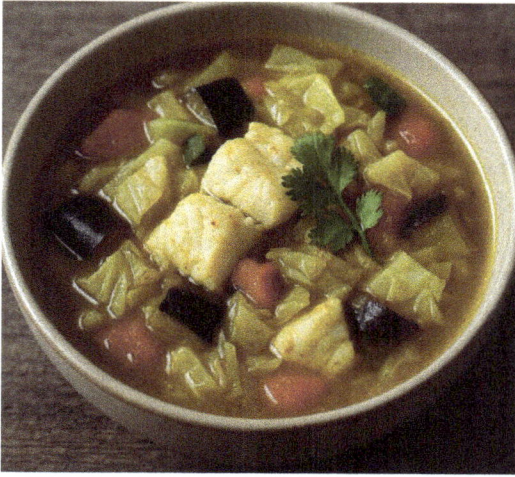

Serves: 1 | **Prep + Cook Time:** ~15–20 minutes | **Calories:** ~140–150 kcal

Ingredients:

- **80g (2.8 oz) white fish fillet** (such as cod, tilapia, snapper), cut into bite-sized chunks
- **1 tablespoon of lime** (or lemon) juice
- **¼ tsp oil (or a splash of water if oil-free)**
- **¼ small onion**, finely chopped
- **1 garlic clove**, minced
- **1/2 medium tomato**, diced
- **1/3 cup eggplant**, diced small
- **2/3 cup green cabbage**, thinly sliced
- *(Total ~1 cup vegetables)*
- **1/2 tsp curry powder**
- **1/4 tsp turmeric** *(optional)*
- **1 cup water or low-sodium broth**
- **Salt and pepper to taste**
- Optional: garnish with fresh cilantro

Instructions:

1. **Marinate the fish in lime (or lemon) juice to remove any fishy odour.**
   Keep it soaked until ready to use. (Lime works better than lemon for this.)

2. **Sauté aromatics to flavour the oil:**
   In a small pot, heat ¼ **tsp oil** over medium heat. Add the **garlic** and **onion**, and sauté for 1–2 minutes until fragrant and slightly golden. This step infuses the oil with flavour.

3. **Add eggplant and cabbage:**
   Stir in the **eggplant** and **cabbage**. Cook for another 2–3 minutes to soften the vegetables.

4. **Add tomato and spices:**
   Add the **diced tomato, curry powder**, and **turmeric**. Stir and cook for 1–2 minutes to allow the spices to bloom.

5. **Add liquid and simmer:**
   Pour in **1 cup water or broth**. Simmer for **5–7 minutes**, until the vegetables are tender.

6. **Add fish and finish:**
   Drain off the lime juice before adding the fish into the soup. Gently add the **white fish** pieces. Simmer for about **2 minutes**, until the fish turns opaque. Do not overcook.

7. **Serve:**
   Season with **salt and pepper**, and garnish with a few drops of **lemon juice** or fresh **cilantro** if desired. Serve hot.

Estimated Nutrition (per serving):
Protein: ~17g | Fat: ~3g | Carbohydrates: ~7g | Fiber: ~2–3g

12.4 Boxing-Day Turkey Veggie Soup – Satiety Starter

This recipe is perfect for the days after Christmas and Thanksgiving, making delicious use of leftover holiday turkey.

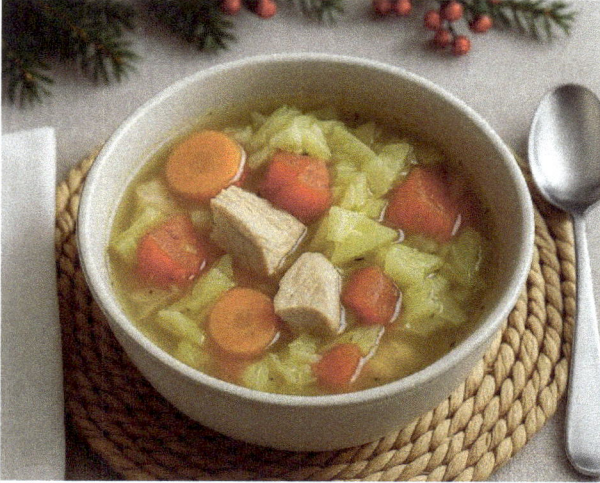

Serves: 1 | **Prep + Cook Time:** ~15–20 minutes | **Calories:** ~135 kcal

Ingredients:

- **50g (1.8 oz) cooked turkey**, shredded or diced
- **¼ teaspoon olive oil**
- **¼ small onion**, finely chopped
- **½ cup carrot**, thinly sliced
- **½ medium tomato**, diced
- **½ cup green cabbage**, thinly sliced
- *(Total vegetables ~1 cup)*
- **1 garlic clove**, minced *(optional)*
- **1 cup water** or low-sodium chicken/turkey broth
- **1/4 tsp dried thyme** or mixed herbs
- **Salt and pepper to taste**
- Optional: squeeze of lemon or garnish with parsley

Instructions:

1. **Sauté aromatics and carrot:**
   In a small pot, heat a splash of water or ¼ tsp oil. Sauté **onion** and **garlic until soften. Then add carrot**. Sauté for 2–3 minutes until starting to soften.

2. **Add tomato and cabbage:**
   Stir in the **tomato** and **cabbage**, and cook for another 2 minutes to release flavour and soften the cabbage slightly.

3. **Add water and simmer:**
   Pour in **1 cup water or broth**. Add **thyme** and simmer for **6–8 minutes**, until vegetables are tender.

4. **Add turkey:**
   Stir in the **turkey** and simmer for just **2–3 minutes** more to warm through.

5. **Season and serve:**
   Add **salt and pepper** to taste. Garnish with **parsley** or a **splash of lemon juice** if desired. Serve hot.

Estimated Nutrition (per serving):

Protein: ~13g | **Fat:** ~4g | **Carbohydrates:** ~8g | **Fiber:** ~2g

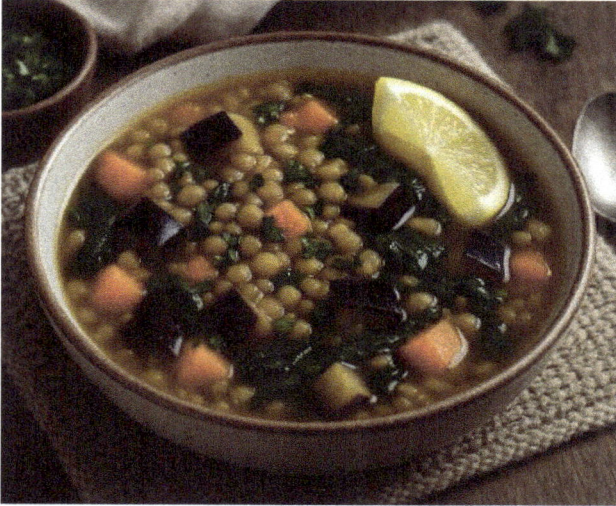

Serves: 1 | **Prep + Cook Time:** ~25 minutes | **Calories:** ~120–130 kcal

Ingredients:

- **25g (0.9 oz) dry red or brown lentils** (~2 tbsp), rinsed
- **¼ teaspoon olive oil**
- **¼ small onion**, finely chopped
- **½ cup carrot**, diced
- **¼ cup eggplant**, diced
- **½ cup spinach** or chopped kale
- **1 garlic clove**, minced
- **1 cup water** or vegetable broth
- **1/4 tsp ground cumin**
- **1/4 tsp ground coriander**
- **Pinch of turmeric or paprika** (optional)
- **Salt and pepper to taste**
- Optional: lemon wedge, fresh parsley or cilantro

Instructions:

1. **Sauté aromatics:**
   In a small pot, sauté the **onion** and **garlic** with a splash of water or ¼ tsp oil for 2 minutes until fragrant.

2. **Add spices and vegetables:**
   Stir in **cumin, coriander,** and **turmeric** (if using). Add **carrot, eggplant** and **lentils**. Sauté lightly for 1 minute to coat with spices.

3. **Simmer:**
   Pour in **1 cup of water or broth**. Bring to a boil, then reduce heat and simmer for 15–20 minutes until lentils and vegetables are tender.

4. **Add greens and finish:**
   Stir in **spinach** and simmer for 1–2 more minutes. Season with **salt and pepper**.

5. **Serve:**
   Garnish with a squeeze of **lemon juice** and **fresh herbs** if desired.

Estimated Nutrition (per serving):

Protein: ~7g | **Fat:** ~1g | **Carbohydrates:** ~18g | **Fiber:** ~5g

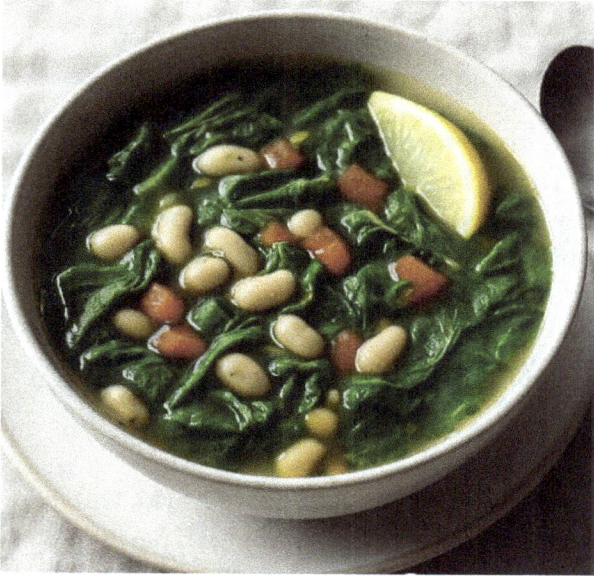

Serves: 1 | **Calories:** ~125–130 kcal | **Prep + Cook Time:** ~15–20 minutes

Ingredients:

- **65g (2.3 oz) cooked white beans** (*e.g., cannellini or navy beans*) (*or use ¼ cup dry beans pre-cooked ahead of time or from a can*)
- **¼ teaspoon olive oil**
- **2 cups fresh spinach**, tightly packed (about 60g)
- **¼ small onion**, chopped
- **1 garlic clove**, minced
- **½ medium tomato**, diced (*optional*)
- **1 cup water** or low-sodium vegetable broth
- **¼ tsp ground cumin**
- **Pinch of turmeric or smoked paprika** (*optional*)
- **Salt and pepper to taste**
- Optional: lemon wedge, chopped parsley

Instructions:

1. **Sauté aromatics:**
   In a small pot, heat a splash of water or ¼ tsp oil. Sauté **onion** and **garlic** for 2–3 minutes until fragrant.

2. **Add beans and simmer:**
   Stir in the **white beans, cumin**, and **turmeric** (if using). Add **1 cup water or broth**, bring to a gentle boil, and simmer for 5 minutes to let flavours meld.

3. **Add spinach and tomato:**
   Stir in the **spinach** and **tomato**. Cook for another 2–3 minutes until the spinach is wilted and soft.

4. **Season and serve:**
   Add **salt and pepper** to taste. Serve warm, with a **squeeze of lemon** and a sprinkle of **fresh herbs** if desired.

Estimated Nutrition (per serving):

Protein: ~7g | **Fat:** ~1g | **Carbohydrates:** ~18g | **Fiber:** ~5g

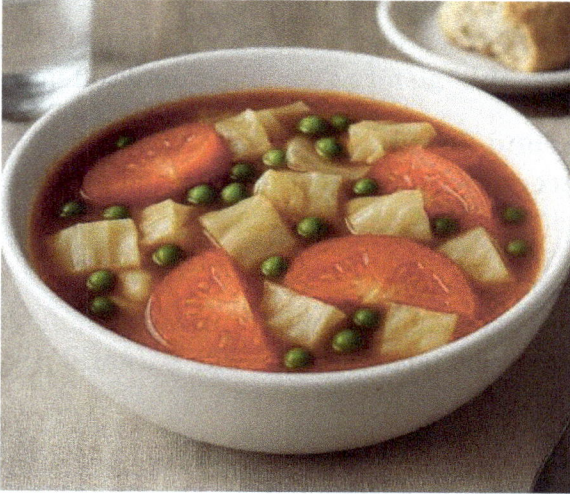

Serves: 1 | **Calories:** ~125–130 kcal | **Prep + Cook Time:** ~15–20 minutes

Ingredients:

- **70g (2.5 oz) cooked/frozen green peas** *(≈ 82 kcal, ~½ cup cooked)*
- **¼ teaspoon olive oil**
- **1 large tomato**, cut to 8 pieces (about 150g)
- **½ cup green cabbage**, shredded
- **¼ cup onion**, chopped
- *(Total vegetables including tomato = ~1 cup)*
- **1 garlic clove**, minced
- **1 cup water** or low-sodium vegetable broth
- **¼ tsp smoked paprika** *(or regular paprika)*
- **Salt and pepper to taste**
- Optional: fresh parsley, basil, or a squeeze of lemon

Instructions:

1. **Sauté aromatics and cabbage:**
   In a small pot, heat a splash of water or ¼ tsp oil. Sauté **onion**, **garlic**, and **cabbage** for 2–3 minutes until softened slightly.

2. **Add peas and liquid:**
   Add the **green peas**, **water or broth**, and **paprika**. Bring to a gentle boil.

3. **Simmer and season:**
   Reduce heat and simmer for **8–10 minutes**, until the soup is rich and vegetables are tender. Season with **salt and pepper** to taste.

4. **Add tomato:**
   Stir in the **chopped tomato** and cook for 2 more minutes, letting the tomato break down slightly.

5. **Serve:**
   Garnish with **herbs or a splash of lemon juice** for brightness if desired.

Estimated Nutrition (per serving):

Protein: ~6g | **Fat:** ~1g | **Carbohydrates:** ~21g | **Fiber:** ~5g

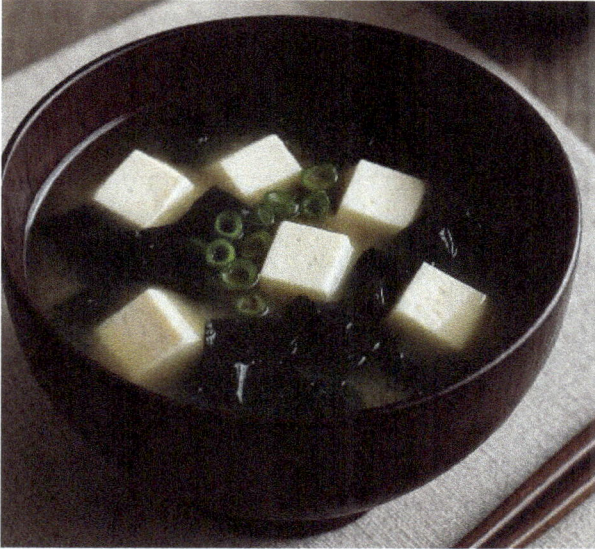

Serves: 1 | **Calories:** ~125 kcal | **Prep + Cook Time:** ~10–15 minutes

Ingredients:

- **60g (2.1 oz) firm tofu,** cubed *(≈ 86 kcal)*

- **5g dried wakame seaweed** *(rehydrates to ~1 cup)*

- **1 tbsp miso paste** *(white or mixed, ~35 kcal)*

- **1 cup water**

- **¼ tsp soy sauce** *(optional, for depth)*

- **1 spring onion,** thinly sliced *(for garnish)*

Instructions:

1. **Rehydrate the seaweed:**
   Soak **5g dried wakame** in water for 5–10 minutes until it expands. Drain and set aside.

2. **Prepare the miso broth:**
   Heat **1 cup of water** in a small saucepan until hot (not boiling). Dissolve **1 tbsp miso paste** in a ladle of hot water, then stir it back into the pot. Keep the heat low to preserve the miso's nutrients.

3. **Add tofu and seaweed:**
   Gently stir in **cubed tofu** and **rehydrated seaweed**. Simmer for 2–3 minutes until warmed through.

4. **Finish and serve:**
   Add **soy sauce** to taste. Garnish with **spring onion** and enjoy warm.

Estimated Nutrition:

Protein: ~10g | **Fat:** ~5g | **Carbohydrates:** ~7g | **Fiber:** ~2g

13 Bonus Chapter: Beyond the Starter – Main Course Soups

You have now learned how powerful a well-designed satiety starter can be. But what comes next matters just as much. To extend the benefits of appetite control and keep hunger at bay, your main meals must also strike the right balance between **volume**, **nutrient density**, and **energy control**.

Hearty Soups for a Light Yet Satisfying Main Meal. Soups are perfect for this. When thoughtfully prepared, they can serve as a full, satisfying meal—warming, comforting, and nutritionally complete.

In this bonus section, I share a simple formula to build your own main course soup, plus a sample recipe to get you started.

13.1 Main Meal Soup Formula

Use the following as a general guide for 1 serving:

- **Protein – choose one of the following:**
    - Lean meat or seafood: 100–120 g (3.5-4.2 oz)
    - Plant-based protein: 1- 1 ½ cup
    - Or a mix: 50 g (1.8 oz) meat + ½ cup plant-based protein
- **Vegetables:** 1–1½ cups firm or leafy vegetables
- **Liquid:** 1 to 1½ cups of broth or water
- **Carbohydrates:** ½ cup cooked rice or other grains, ¾ medium potato, 2/3 cup pasta loosely packed,
- **Fat:** ½ teaspoon of oil or cream (optional)
- **Flavour:** herbs, spices, garlic, or onion for aroma and taste

Chicken Pasta Soup

Approx. 392 kcal | 37.5g protein

Ingredients:

- 100g (3.5oz) cooked skinless chicken breast (shredded or diced)
- 75g (2.6oz) cooked whole wheat pasta (small shapes like macaroni or ditalini)
- ½ cup chopped carrot
- ½ cup chopped cabbage
- ½ medium tomato
- ½ small onion, finely diced
- 1 clove garlic, minced
- 1 cup low-sodium chicken broth
- 1 teaspoon olive oil (for sautéing)
- Salt, pepper, parsley to taste

Instructions:

1. Sauté the onion and garlic in olive oil over medium heat until fragrant.

2. Add chopped carrot and cabbage, and stir for 2–3 minutes.

3. Pour in the broth and bring to a boil.

4. Add cooked pasta, tomato and chicken. Reduce heat and simmer for about 2 minutes.

5. Season to taste & garnish with fresh parsley before serving.

When substituting meat with plant-based protein, you may need a larger quantity to match the same protein content. However, this increase often comes with additional calories—so it is wise to reduce the amount of carbohydrates in the meal to maintain balance. Here are the amount of plant-based proteins to use:

Plant-Based Protein (Cooked)	Protein (per 100g)	Amount Needed to Match 100g meat (cooked)
Lentils	~9g	~300g (about 1⅓ cups)
White beans	~8g	~340g (about 1½ cups)
Chickpeas	~8.5g	~320g (about 1⅓ cups)
Tofu (firm)	~12g	~225g (about ¾ block)
Tempeh	~19g	~140g
Edamame	~11g	~245g

White Bean Pasta Soup

Approx. 401 kcal | 19.5g protein

Ingredients:

- 1 cup (160 g / 5.6 oz) cooked white beans (to match protein content of meat)

- 40 g (1.4 oz) cooked whole wheat pasta

- ½ cup chopped carrot

- ½ cup chopped cabbage

- ½ medium tomato

- ½ small onion, finely diced

- 1 clove garlic, minced

- 1 cup water or low-sodium vegetable broth

- ½ teaspoon olive oil (for sautéing)

- Salt, pepper, parsley to taste

Instructions:

1. Heat olive oil in a pot and sauté the onion and garlic until soft.

2. Add carrot and cabbage, and stir for 2–3 minutes.

3. Pour in the broth, bring to a boil, then reduce to a simmer.

4. Stir in the cooked beans, tomato and cooked pasta. Simmer for 5–7 minutes.

5. Adjust seasoning and garnish with parsley.

These soups deliver a satisfying, slow-digesting meal that supports satiety while keeping calories in check. It is perfect for lunch, a light dinner, or meal prep for the week.

Want more? In my next book, I will share a collection of **main meal soups** inspired by different cuisines, all nutritionally balanced for weight and wellness.

14 My Future Books and Final Words

Knowledge gains meaning when it helps others rise, thrive, and transform—and that is what drives me to continue this series on Exercise and Nutrition for Health and Weight Management.

In my upcoming Books, I will continue exploring health questions that have puzzled many—including myself—and uncover what peer-reviewed research really says. Most importantly, I will share these insights with you in a way that is practical, clear, and actionable.

Next, I will pick up where we left off: exploring what a truly healthy diet looks like—one that not only supports **sustainable weight loss**, but also promotes **lifelong vitality**. I will introduce the different effective forms of exercise and their unique benefits. These can be **seamlessly integrated with satiety strategies** to help curb overeating and reclaim control over your health—one powerful habit at a time.

If you are searching for a way of eating that is both **healthy and sustainable**, the next book is written with you in mind.

Because real, lasting change does not come from extremes—it comes from balance. The pre-meal satiety strategies you have just learned are a powerful start. But when paired with a nourishing daily routine that satisfies and supports your goals, they become truly transformative.

That is the focus of this next book: to guide you toward food choices that are not only effective but genuinely empowering—for the long run, and for the life you deserve.

While You Wait for the Next Book...

I write my Books and do the research myself. While AI helps speed things up, I carefully check every detail to ensure the information is as accurate and current as possible. That is why my next book will take time—I want to get it right. If you are eager to take action now—to achieve and maintain a healthier weight—you do not have to wait. You can begin today:

1. **Start with pre-meal satiety starters.** Use light, well-planned starters to gently curb your appetite and reduce calorie intake during your main meals—especially those meals where you tend to overeat.

2. **Choose foods that nourish and satisfy.** Focus on **lower energy density** foods that are **rich in essential nutrients**. Fill your plate with a tasty variety of colourful non-starchy vegetables, fresh fruits, and lean proteins. These foods not only support weight management but also nourish your body. Cut back on high-calorie foods, especially those you eat out of habit rather than enjoyment. Use lower-energy options like low-fat, but compare labels for added sugars and total calories.

3. **Practice meal sequencing:** start meals with foods rich in water such as plain water, low-calorie beverages or chunky soup, **follow by fibre—** like salads or lower GI fruits—followed by **protein-rich dishes**, while **delaying carbohydrates and fats to the last**, can help:

   o Increase **satiety per calorie** (helping you feel full with fewer calories)

   o Reduce **blood sugar spikes** after meals

   o Lower **oxidative stress and inflammation**

   This strategy is also supported by research. A review by Shapira (2019) echoes these findings, highlighting the value of thoughtful meal sequencing.

4. **Dealing with excess food and dessert.** Give your body a chance to catch up—wait until you have finished your main meal before deciding on dessert. You might be surprised to find you no longer need it. And if you feel full before your plate is empty, simply stop eating. Do not force yourself to finish the food. You can always store the rest for another meal. As your appetite adjusts, start preparing and serving less food, especially the high-calorie items.

5. **Rethink your snacking habits.** Frequent snacking can sneak in extra calories and stimulate your appetite more than you realise. How often have you opened a bag of snacks intending to have just one... and found yourself finishing the whole packet? To avoid this, buy smaller, lower-caloric portions and healthier options, keep them out of easy reach, and most importantly—pause and ask yourself if you are truly hungry.

6. **Stay well hydrated.** Aim for around 8 glasses of fluid / water a day, inclusive of your non-alcoholic beverages and soups. Our bodies can sometimes confuse thirst with hunger—yes, it really can be that subtle. Keeping well hydrated not only supports metabolism and digestion but may also help prevent unnecessary snacking. But avoid sugar-laden soft drinks and beverages.

7. **Stay physically active doing what you love.** Whether it is dancing, walking, tidying your space, or a burst of cardio, movement lifts your mood and helps burn excess fat. **If there are times you are prone to snacking, use those moments to get moving**—you will feel better, stronger, and more in control.

Final words...

Thank you for reading. I hope this Book has given you a clearer understanding of how **pre-meal satiety starters** and **low energy density foods** can support appetite control and foster healthier eating habits.

I look forward to connecting with you again in my next Book, where we will continue exploring practical, evidence-based strategies for healthy lasting change.

Until then—**stay curious, stay nourished, and take good care.**

If this Book has helped or inspired you in any way, I would be truly grateful if you could leave a rating or review on **Amazon,** and Goodreads if you are a member or librarian. Your feedback not only supports my work, but also helps others discover tools that may support their own journey. Whether you share how it helped or offer thoughtful suggestions, your voice is valued—and appreciated.

A Prayer for the Journey:

As you finish this book, may this prayer encourage and guide you...

Holy God in Heaven,

For readers who are struggling with obesity, excess weight, and the toll it takes on their health and spirit, I pray You will bring comfort, strength, and renewed hope to those who seek change.

I pray that this Book may serve as a helpful guide—offering understanding, practical wisdom, and encouragement to those in need. May it point them toward healing, both in body and in heart.

I ask this through Christ, our Saviour.

Amen.

Acknowledgement

This book would not have been possible without the support, guidance, and contributions of many individuals and researchers.

First and foremost, I want to thank you, the reader. This book is written for those seeking practical ways to manage overeating and take control of their appetite. Your willingness to explore new strategies and your commitment to improving your health are the reasons this book exists. I hope the insights shared here help you make positive, lasting changes.

I am also grateful to the many researchers whose work is referenced throughout these pages. Your dedication to studying appetite control, satiety responses, and pre-meal strategies provided the scientific basis for this book. Your efforts in advancing knowledge in this field have been instrumental, and I deeply appreciate your contributions to the field of science.

A heartfelt thank you to my family and friends who offered invaluable feedback and encouragement throughout the writing process. I am especially grateful to my husband and family members temporarily living with us, who took on much of the housework and cooking so I could concentrate on this project. Your unwavering support and practical help made all the difference—not to mention your willingness to be my enthusiastic recipe-taste-testers along the way.

Last but not least, I would like to thank my former dissertation supervisor, Professor Stephen Fallows, and second examiner, Mrs Mary Cotterell, at the University of Chester. Although it has been years since I graduated, I remain grateful for your thoughtful guidance and constructive feedback during my Master degree's research in Exercise and Nutrition Science. Your support helped shape the foundations of this book, and your encouragement continues to inspire my work.

Thank you to everyone who made this book possible and to all those who will benefit from it.

References

List of Preload Studies

Ahn, C. H., Min, K. W., Hong, J. Y., Cho, Y. M., & Chung, S. S. (2019). Premeal consumption of a protein-enriched, dietary fiber-fortified bar decreases total energy intake in healthy individuals. *Diabetes & Metabolism Journal, 43*(6), 808–818. https://doi.org/10.4093/dmj.2018.0122

Almiron-Roig E, Flores SY, Drewnowski A (2004). No difference in satiety or in subsequent energy intakes between a beverage and a solid food. *Physiology and Behavior.* 82: 671-677

Anderson GH, Woodend D (2003). Consumption of sugars and the regulation of short-term satiety and food intake. *American Journal of Clinical Nutrition.* 78:843S-9S

Caton SJ, Ball M, Ahern A, Hetherington MM (2004). Dose-independent effects of alcohol on appetite and food intake. *Physiology and Behavior.* 81,1, P51-58.

Cecil JE, Francis J, Read NW (1999). Comparison of the effects of a high-fat and high-carbohydrate soup delivered orally and intragastrically on gastric emptying, appetite, and eating behaviour. *Physiology and Behavior.* Aug;67(2):299-306.

de Graaf C, Hulshof T (1996). Effects of weight and energy content of preloads on subsequent appetite and food intake. *Appetite.* Apr;26(2):139-51.

Flood-Obbagy, J. E., & Rolls, B. J. (2009). The effect of fruit in different forms on energy intake and satiety at a meal. *Appetite, 52*(2), 416–422. https://doi.org/10.1016/j.appet.2008.12.001

Gray R, French S, Robinson T, Yeomans M (2002). Dissociation of the effects of preload volume and energy content on subjective appetite and food intake. *Physiology and Behavior.* May 1;76(1):57-64.

Gray RW, French SJ, Robinson TM, Yeomans MR (2003). Increasing Preload volume with water reduces rated appetite but not food intake in healthy men even with minimum delay between preload and test meal. *Nutritional Neuroscience.* Vol 6 (1) pp29-37.

Himaya A, Louis-Sylvestre J (1998). The effect of soup on satiation. *Appetite.* Apr;30(2):199-210.

Holt SHA, Sandona N and Brand-Miller (2000). The effects of sugar-free vs sugar-rich beverages on feelings of fullness and subsequent food intake. *International Journal of Food Sciences and Nutrition.* 51, 59-71.

Hulshof T, De Graaf C, Weststrate JA (1993). The effects of preloads varying in physical state and fat content on satiety and energy intake. Appetite. Dec;21(3):273-86.

Jeong, J. N. (2018). Effect of pre-meal water consumption on energy intake and satiety in non-obese young adults. *Clinical Nutrition Research, 7*(4), 291–296. https://doi.org/10.7762/cnr.2018.7.4.291

Johnston, C. S., Foreyt, J. P., & Poston, W. S. C. (2013). The effect of peanut and grain bar preloads on postmeal satiety, glycemia, and weight loss in healthy individuals. *Nutrition Journal, 12*, 17. https://doi.org/10.1186/1475-2891-12-17

Johnstone AM, Shannon E, Whybrow S, Reid CA, Stubbs RJ (2000). Altering the temporal distribution of energy intake with isoenergetically dense foods given a snack does not affect total daily energy intake in normal-weight men. *British Journal of Nutrition*. 83, 7-14

Kim JY, Kissileff HR (1996). The effect of social setting on response to a preloading manipulation in non-obese women and men. *Appetite*. Aug;27(1):25-40.

King, J. A., Wasse, L. K., Ewens, J., Crystallis, K., Emmanuel, J., & Batterham, R. L. (2022). Effects of pre-meal whey protein consumption on acute food intake and energy balance over a 48-hour period. *Appetite, 168*, 105741. https://doi.org/10.1016/j.appet.2021.105741

Lappalainen R, Mennen L, Weert v, Mykkanen H (1993). Drinking water with a meal: a simple method of coping with feelings of hunger, satiety and desire to eat. *European Journal of Clinical Nutrition*. 47, 815-819

Lee, A. S., Ryu, J., Han, Y., Kim, J., & Yoon, J. (2021). Effects of unsweetened preloads and preloads sweetened with caloric or low-/no-calorie sweeteners on subsequent energy intakes: A systematic review and meta-analysis. *Nutrients, 13*(2), 569. https://doi.org/10.3390/nu13020569

Luscombe-Marsh, N. D., Seimon, R. V., Bollmeyer, E., Wishart, J. M., Wittert, G. A., Horowitz, M., Bellon, M., & Feinle-Bisset, C. (2013). Acute effects of oral preloads with increasing energy density on gastric emptying, gut hormone release, thermogenesis and energy intake in overweight and obese men. *Asia Pacific Journal of Clinical Nutrition, 22*(3), 380–390.

Oesch, S., Ruegg, C., Fischer, K., D'Alessio, D. A., Tappy, L., & Schutz, Y. (2005). Effect of a protein preload on food intake and satiety with and without intraduodenal lipid perfusion in healthy male subjects. *American Journal of Clinical Nutrition, 82*(2), 366–373. https://doi.org/10.1093/ajcn/82.2.366

Parretti, H. M., Aveyard, P., Blannin, A., Clifford, S. J., Coleman, S. J., Roalfe, A., & Daley, A. J. (2015). Efficacy of water preloading before main meals as a strategy for weight loss in primary care patients with obesity: A randomized controlled trial. *Obesity, 23*(9), 1785–1791. https://doi.org/10.1002/oby.21167

Parretti, H., Aveyard, P., Blannin, A., Clifford, S., Coleman, S., Roalfe, A., & Daley, A. (2015). Efficacy of water preloading before main meals as a strategy for weight loss in primary care patients with obesity. *Obesity*, *23*(9), 1785–1791. https://doi.org/10.1002/oby.21167

Poppitt SD, McCormack D, Buffenstein R (1998). Short-term effects of macronutrient preloads on appetite and energy intake in lean women. *Physiology and Behavior*. Jun 1;64(3):279-85.

Porrini M, Crovetti R, Testolin G, Silva S (1995). Evaluation of satiety sensations and food intake after different preloads. *Appetite*. Aug;25(1):17-30.

Porrini M, Santangelo A, Crovetti R, Riso P, Testolin G, Blundell JE (1997). Weight, protein, fat, and timing of preloads affect food intake. *Physiology and Behavior*. Sep;62(3):563-70.

Raben A, Agerholm-Larsen L, Flint A, Holst J, Astrup A (2003). Meals with similar energy densities but rich in protein, fat, carbohydrate, or alcohol have different effects on energy expenditure and substrate metabolism but not on appetite and energy intake. American Journal of Clinical Nutrition. 77:91-100

Rodin J (1990). Comparative effects of fructose, aspartame, glucose, and water preloads on calorie and macronutrient intake. American Journal of Clinical Nutrition. Mar;51(3):428-35.

Rolls BJ, Bell EA, Thorwart ML (1999). Water incorporated into a food but not served with a food decreases energy intake in lean women. *American Journal of Clinical Nutrition*. 70:448-55

Rolls BJ, Bell EA, Waugh BA (2000). Increasing the volume of a food by incorporating air affects satiety in men. *American Journal of Clinical Nutrition*. 72:361-8.

Rolls BJ, Castellanos VH, Halford JC, Kilara A, Panyam D, Pelkman, Smith GP, Thorwart ML (1998). Volume of food consumed affects satiety in men. *American Journal of Clinical Nutrition*. 67:1170-77.

Rolls BJ, Kim S, McNelis AL, Fischman MW, Foltin RW, Moran TH (1991). Time course of effects of preloads high in fat or carbohydrate on food intake and hunger ratings in humans. *American Journal of Physiology*. Apr;260(4 Pt 2):R756-63.

Rolls BJ, Kim-Harris S, Fischman MW, Foltin RW, Moran TH, Stoner SA (1994). Satiety after preloads with different amounts of fat and carbohydrate: implications for obesity. *American Journal of Clinical Nutrition*. Oct;60(4):476-87.

Rolls BJ, Roe LS (2002). Effect of the volume of liquid food infused intragastrically on satiety in women. *Physiology and Behavior*. 76 (2002) 623-631.

Rouhani, M. H., Surkan, P. J., & Azadbakht, L. (2017). The effect of preload/meal energy density on energy intake in a subsequent meal: A systematic review and meta-analysis. *Eating Behaviors, 26,* 6–15. https://doi.org/10.1016/j.eatbeh.2016.12.011

Smith, K., Read, L., Chan, A., Clegg, M., & Pacy, P. (2021). Effects of pre-meal whey protein consumption on postprandial glucose, gut hormones, and gastric emptying in lean and centrally obese adult males. *Frontiers in Endocrinology, 12,* 696977. https://doi.org/10.3389/fendo.2021.696977

Spiegel TA, Hubert CD, Fried H, Peikin SR, Siegel JA, Zeiger LS (1997). Contribution of gastric and postgastric feedback to satiation and satiety in women. Physiology and Behavior. Nov;62(5):1125-36.

Spiegel TA, Kaplan JM, Alavi A, Kim PS, Tse KK (1993). Effects of soup preloads on gastric emptying and fullness ratings following an egg sandwich meal. Physiology and Behavior. Sep;56(3):571-5.

Van de Ven ML, Westerterp-Plantenga MS, Wouters L, Saris WH (1994). Effects of liquid preloads with different fructose/fibre concentrations on subsequent food intake and ratings of hunger in women. *Appetite.* Oct;23(2):139-46.

Van Walleghen, E. L., Orr, J. S., Gentile, C. L., & Davy, B. M. (2007). Pre-meal water consumption reduces meal energy intake in older but not younger subjects. *Obesity, 15*(1), 93–99. https://doi.org/10.1038/oby.2007.506

Westerterp-Plantenga, MS, Verwegen CRT (1999). The appetizing effect of an aperitif in overweight and normal weight humans. *American Journal of Clinical Nutrition.* Feb; 69:205-12

Woodend DM, Anderson GH (2001). Effect of sucrose and safflower oil preloads on short term appetite and food intake of young men. *Appetite.* Dec;37(3):185-95.

Yeomans MR, Lartamo S, Procter EL, Lee MD, Gray RW (2001). The actual, but not labeled, fat content of a soup preload alters short-term appetite in healthy men. *Physiology and Behavior.* 73 (2001) 533-540

Yeomans MR, Lee MD, Gray RW, French SJ (2001). Effects of test-meal palatability on compensatory eating following disguised fat and carbohydrate preloads. *International Journal of Obesity and Related Metabolic Disorder.* Aug;25(8):1215-24.

Yeomans MR, Phillips MF (2001). Failure to Reduce Short-term Appetite Following Alcohol is independent of beliefs about the presence of alcohol. *Nutritional Neuroscience.* Vol 5 (2) pp 131-139.

Other References

Accinelli, R. A., & León-Abarca, J. A. (2019). Five or more hours of smartphone usage per day may increase obesity. *American College of Cardiology*. https://www.acc.org/about-acc/press-releases/2019/07/25/14/23/five-or-more-hours-of-smartphone-usage-per-day-may-increase-obesity

Aitman TJ (2003). Genetic Medicine and Obesity, *New England Journal of Medicine*, Volume 348:2138-2139 May 22 Number 21

Bakour, C., Shankar, P., & Nieto, F. J. (2022). Association between screen time and obesity in U.S. adolescents: A national study. *Preventive Medicine Reports, 27*, 101800. https://doi.org/10.1016/j.pmedr.2022.101800

Batterham RL, Cohen MA, Ellis SM, Le Roux CW, Withers DJ, Frost GS, Ghatei MA, Bloom SR. Inhibition of Food Intake in Obese Subjects by Peptide YY3–36 *New England Journal Medicine,* 349:941-948, Sep 4, 2003.

Bellisle, F., Drewnowski, A., Anderson, G. H., Westerterp-Plantenga, M., & Martin, C. K. (2012). Sweetness, satiation, and satiety. *The Journal of Nutrition, 142*(6), 1149S–1154S. https://doi.org/10.3945/jn.111.149583

Benelam, B. (2009). Satiation, satiety and their effects on eating behaviour. *Nutrition Bulletin, 34*(2), 126–173. https://doi.org/10.1111/j.1467-3010.2009.01753.x

Brunstrom, J. M. (2014). Mind over platter: pre-meal planning and the control of meal size in humans. *International Journal of Obesity, 38*(S1), S9–S12. https://doi.org/10.1038/ijo.2014.83

Delargy HJ, O'Sullivan KR, Fletcher RJ, Blundell JE (1997). Effects of amount and type of dietary fibre (soluble and insoluble) on short-term control of appetite. *International Journal of Food Sciences and Nutrition.* Jan;48(1):67-77.

Deurenberg, Deurenberg-Yap M, Foo LF, Schmidt G, Wang J (2003). Differences in body composition between Singapore Chinese, Beijing Chinese and Dutch children, *International Journal of Obesity*, March, Volume 57, Number 3, Pages 405-409

Deurenberg-Yap M, Chew SK, Lin VFP, Tan BY, van Staveren WA, Deurenberg P (2001). Relationships between indices of obesity and its co-morbidities in multi-ethnic Singapore, *International Journal of Obesity*, October, Volume 25, Number 10, Pages 1554-1562

Deurenberg-Yap M, Schmidt G, van Staveren WA, Deurenberg P (2000). The paradox of low body mass index and high body fat percentage among Chinese, Malays and Indians in Singapore, *International Journal of Obesity*, August, Volume 24, Number 8, Pages 1011-1017

106

Fleur SE, Zwaal EM (2014) Satietion, Satiety and the Control of Food Intake. *ScienceDirect, Woodhead Publishing Series in Food Science, Technology and Nutrition 2013, Pages 55-74*

Freedman MR, King J, Kennedy E (2001). Popular Diets: A Scientific Review. *Obesity Research,* Vol. 9 Suppl. 1 March.

Fu WPC, Lee HC, Ng CJ, Tay YKD, Kau CY, Seow CJ, Siak JK, Hong CY (2003). Screening for childhood obesity: international vs population-specific definitions. Which is more appropriate? *International Journal of Obesity*, September, Volume 27, Number 9, Pages 1121-1126

Garrow JS, James WPT (1998). *Human Nutrition and Dietetics* (9th ed). Churchill Livingstone, UK.

Jerome P. Kassirer and Marcia Angell (1998). Losing Weight — An Ill-Fated New Year's Resolution, *New England Journal of Medicine*, Volume 338:52-54 January 1, No 1

Kassirer JP, Angell M (1998). Losing weight – an ill-fated new year's resolution. *The New England Journal of Medicine,* Volume 338:52-54, January

Lahti-Koski M, Pietinen P, Heliovaara M, Vartiainen E (2002). Associations of body mass index and obesity with physical activity, food choices, alcohol intake and smoking in the 1982-1997 FINRISK studies. *The American Journal of Clinical Nutrition,* Vol 75, No 5, 809-817, May.

Lim SC, Tan BY, Chew SK, Tan CE (2002). The relationship between insulin resistance and cardiovascular risk factors in overweight/obese non-diabetic Asian adults: the 1992 *Singapore National Health Survey, Journal of Obesity,* November, Volume 26, Number 11, Pages 1511-1516

Lindpaintner K (1995). Finding an Obesity Gene — A Tale of Mice and Man, *New England Journal of Medicine*, Volume 332:679-680 March 9, Number 10

Llewellyn CH, Trzaskowski M, Jaarsveld CHM (2014) Satiety Mechanisms in Genetic Risk of Obesity, *JAMA April*

Marmonier C, Chapelot D, Louis-Sylvestre J (2000). Effects of macronutrient content and energy density of snacks consumed in a satiety state on the onset of the next meal. *Appetite*. Apr;34(2):161-8.

McCrory MA, Suen VMM, Roberts B (2002). Biobehavioral Influences on Energy Intake and Adult Weight Gain, The American Society for Nutritional Sciences *Journal of Nutrition*. 132:3830S-3834S, December.

Nesti, L., Mengozzi, A., & Tricò, D. (2019). Impact of Nutrient Type and Sequence on Glucose Tolerance: Physiological Insights and Therapeutic Implications, *Frontiers in Endocrinology*, *10*, 144. https://doi.org/10.3389/fendo.2019.00144

Oesch, S., Degen, L., & Beglinger, C. (2005). Effect of a protein preload on food intake and satiety feelings in response to duodenal fat perfusions in healthy male subjects. American Journal of Physiology-Regulatory, Integrative and Comparative Physiology, 289(4), R1042–R1047. https://doi.org/10.1152/ajpregu.00039.2005

Pearcey SM, Castro JM (2002). Food intake and meal patterns of weight-stable and weight-gaining persons, *American Journal of Clinical Nutrition*, Vol. 76, No. 1, 107-112, July

Prentice AM, Jebb SA (1995). Obesity in Britain: gluttony or sloth? *British Medical Journal*; 311:437-439 (12 August)

Rakha, A., Mehak, F., Shabbir, M. A., Arslan, M., Ranjha, M. M. A. N., Ahmed, W., Socol, C. T., Rusu, A. V., Hassoun, A., & Aadil, R. M. (2022). Insights into the constellating drivers of satiety impacting dietary patterns and lifestyle. *Frontiers in Nutrition*, 9, Article 1010817. https://doi.org/10.3389/fnut.2022.1010817

Read N, French S, Cunningham K (1994). The role of the gut in regulating food intake in man. *Nutrition Reviews*, Vol 52, No 1, January

Ristow M., Müller-Wieland D., Pfeiffer A., Krone W., Kahn C. R. (1998) Obesity Associated with a Mutation in a Genetic Regulator of Adipocyte Differentiation, *New England Journal of Medicine,* 1998; 339:953-959, Oct 1

Roberts SB, Williamson DF (2002). Causes of Adult Weight Gain, Symposium: Adult Weight Gain: Causes and Implications, *The American Society for Nutritional Sciences Journal of Nutrition* 132:3824S-3825S, December

Robinson, E., Khuttan, M., McFarland-Lesser, I., Patel, Z., & Jones, A. (2022). Calorie reformulation: A systematic review and meta-analysis examining the effect of manipulating food energy density on daily energy intake. *International Journal of Behavioral Nutrition and Physical Activity,* 19(48). https://doi.org/10.1186/s12966-022-01287-z

Shapira, N. (2019). The metabolic concept of meal sequence vs. satiety: Glycemic and oxidative responses with reference to inflammation risk, protective principles, and Mediterranean diet. *Nutrients,* 11(10), 2373. https://doi.org/10.3390/nu11102373

Stensel DJ, Lin FP, Nevill AM (2001). Resting metabolic rate in obese and nonobese Chinese Singaporean boys aged 13–15 y, *American Journal of Clinical Nutrition*, Vol. 74, No. 3, 369-373, September

Stribițcaia, E., Evans, C. E. L., Gibbons, C., Blundell, J. E., & Sarkar, A. (2020). Food texture influences on satiety: Systematic review and meta-analysis. *Scientific Reports, 10*(1), 12929. https://doi.org/10.1038/s41598-020-69868-2

Stribiţcaia, E., Evans, C. E. L., Gibbons, C., Blundell, J., & Sarkar, A. (2020). Food texture influences on satiety: Systematic review and meta-analysis. *Scientific Reports*, *10*, Article 12929. https://doi.org/10.1038/s41598-020-69778-z

Stubbs RJ, van Wyk MC, Johnstone AM, Harbron CG (1996). Breakfasts high in protein, fat or carbohydrate: effect on within-day appetite and energy balance. *European Journal of Clinical Nutrition.* Jul;50(7):409-17.

Szalanczy AM, Chuang-Key CC, Woods LCS (2022) Genetic variation in satiety signaling and hypothalamic inflammation: merging fields for the study of obesity, *The Journal of Nutritional Biochemistry, Volume 101, March 2022, 108928*

World Health Organization (WHO). (2024). *World health statistics 2024: Monitoring health for the SDGs, sustainable development goals*. World Health Organization. https://iris.who.int/bitstream/handle/10665/376869/9789240094703-eng.pdf

World Health Organization (WHO). (2024, March 1). *One in eight people are now living with obesity – WHO and partners call for action.* https://www.who.int/news/item/01-03-2024-one-in-eight-people-are-now-living-with-obesity

World Health Organization Regional Office for Europe. (2022). *WHO European regional obesity report 2022.* https://www.who.int/europe/publications/i/item/9789289057738

Secondary References

Anderson GH & Moore SE (2004) Dietary proteins in the regulation of food intake and body weight in humans. *Journal of Nutrition* **134**: S974–9 (cited by Benelam, 2009)

World Health Organization. Obesity: prevention and managing the global epidemic. *Report of a WHO Consultation on Obesity*, WHO/NUT/NCD/98.1. WHO: Geneva; 1998.

Appendix A: The Science Behind This Book

This Book is based on a **Master's dissertation in Exercise and Nutrition Science** submitted to the University of Chester. The original research followed a **systematic review approach**, carefully analysing existing studies on preloading and appetite control.

To keep the content **up-to-date and relevant**, newer research findings have been incorporated, ensuring you get the most current insights backed by science.

For those who love the details, the full research methodology is outlined below. But if you are just here for the practical takeaways—feel free to skip ahead and dive into the main content!

I. Research Methodology used in the Original Dissertation

How the Research Was Selected

To ensure the most relevant and credible findings, a careful selection process was used. Only English-language studies were included, and research was sourced from publicly available abstracts found online through scientific journals and search engines.

Once identified, full articles were obtained through purchases, library collections in Singapore (where I was located at that time), or direct requests from the authors. This thorough approach helped compile the most valuable insights on preloading.

Here is how the selection process unfolded:

1.   An online search on the following key websites and search engines:

•   PubMed (www.ncbi.nlm.nih.gov)

•   British Medical Journal (www.bmj.com). Please see 4 below for the list of journals selected for search under BMJ (British Medical Journal) search engine.

•   National University of Singapore Library (http://linc.nus.edu.sg/)

•   Search engines:

i.   www.scirus.com

ii.   www.scholar.google.com

2.   The websites of the publications where research articles have been found are also searched online. These websites include:

- Elsevier Author Gateway (http://authors.elsevier.com):

i.   Appetite

ii.   Physiology and Behavior

- American Journal of Clinical Nutrition (http://ww.ajcn.org)

- Nature Publishing Group (http://www.nature.com)

i.   European Journal of Clinical Nutrition

ii.   International Journal of Obesity and Related Metabolic Disorder

- Taylor and Francis Group (http://www.tandf.co.uk/journals/online.asp):

i.   International Journal of Food Sciences and Nutrition

ii.   Nutritional Neuroscience

3.   For every relevant article found, searches were also extended to the related links in PubMed and for the newer articles which have cited the article found if these are given in the online articles or abstract.

4.   As the effects of preload could affect food intake through physiological, biochemical, hormonal, cognitive or metabolic pathways, all publications covering researches on nutrition, endocrinology, metabolism, obesity, physiology, sports medicine, biochemistry, genetics, gastro-intestinal and general medicine are included in the search. The list of publications included in the BMJ search are as follows:

- American Journal of Clinical Nutrition

- American Journal of Physiology – Endocrinology and Metabolism

- American Journal of Physiology – Gastrointestinal and Liver Physiology

- American Journal of Sports Medicine

- BMJ (British Medical Journal)

- British Journal of Sports Medicine

- Clinical Diabetes

- Endocrine Reviews

- Endocrinology

- European Journal of Biochemistry
- Genome Research
- Genetics
- Human Molecular Genetics
- Health
- Heart
- The FASEB Journal
- Focus
- Gut
- JAMA (Journal of American Medical Association)
- Journal of Applied Physiology
- Journal of Chemical Endocrinology and Metabolism
- Journal of Cognitive Neuroscience
- Journal of General Physiology
- Journal of Heredity
- Journal of Lipid Research
- Journal of Nutrition
- Journal of Neuroscience
- Journal of Neurophysiology
- Journal of the American College of Nutrition
- The Journal of Physiology
- Journal Watch Gastroenterology
- Journal Watch (General)
- Journal Watch Neurology
- Molecular Endocrinology
- Neurology

- New England Journal of Medicine

- Obesity Research

- Physiological Genomics

- Physiological Reviews

- Physiology

- Postgraduate Medical Journal

- Science

II. Keywords used for Search

The following sequence of searches are used on the titles and abstracts and if this selection option is not available (as in Scirus and Google), then the entire document is selected.

1. First the search starts with preload

2. If the search yields over 300 articles and the results yield less than 10%, (an arbitrary number of half is selected as a gauge), of relevant articles, the search has been refined with:

    a. preload AND energy

    b. preload AND appetite

    c. preload AND satiety

3. The search in 2 still yields over 300 articles, the search bas been refined with:

    a. preload AND energy AND appetite AND satiety

For most of the publications websites, searches stops at 1. preload. But with the search engines under PubMed and BMJ, the search combination for 2 has to be used. And with the general web search engines, Scirus and Google, the search combination 3 has to be used.

III. Researches were found primarily published in the following publications:

- American Journal of Clinical Nutrition

- Appetite

- Physiology and Behavior

Isolated articles are also found in the following:

- International Journal of Food Sciences and Nutrition

- Nutritional Neuroscience

- European Journal of Clinical Nutrition

- International Journal of Obesity and Related Metabolic Disorder

- American Journal of Clinical Nutrition

- American Journal of Physiology

A search is made of the above publications online for their research papers using the keyword 'preload' to make sure that the search is exhausted. Any related links were also looked into to help in the search. References made to older papers were also checked up. Searches were also made into articles that referenced cited these papers that were found.

A screening was made of the abstracts or of the full articles if available free online and researches included in the reviews were those made into the effects of preload on energy intake and studying the individual responses to:

a.   macronutrient contents

b.   energy level

c.   time effect

d.   weight or volume

e.   physical state of preload

f.   behavioural differences between different subject groups

Once the research papers are selected, a search of the full articles if it is not available free online were made through one or more of the following ways:

a.   Search of local libraries including that of the National University of Singapore libraries including that of the Medical Library and Central Library.

b.   Search through the University College Chester online resources on IBIS. (http://ibis.chester.ac.uk/)

c.   Assistance of Prof Stephen Fallows who also helped in the search for the full articles which could not be located from the above search.

d.   A purchase is made of the articles online when it is not available in hardcopy from the local libraries or not free from online sources.

e.   A request from the authors themselves if contact information of the authors is available. Requests were made to Drs Rolls and Yeomans for their articles which cannot be located from the above sources and they have kindly forwarded through the email.

A summary of the articles was made based on the following information extracted from the published studies:

1.   Objectives of the study

2.   Number of Subjects

3.   Who were the subjects?

4.   Location of the studies

5.   Investigations: What preload effects were investigated?

6.   Tests: How was the test conducted?

7.   Measures: What measures were made in the study?

8.   Results: What were the key results and findings?

9.   Conclusions of the Study

IV.   Subject (Research) Selection and Exclusion

The effects of the preload examined are:

a.   macronutrient contents

b.   energy level

c.   time effect

d.   weight or volume

e.   physical state of preload

f.   behavioural differences between different subject groups

A critical appraisal was made of the published research and researches. Those that are included in this study are those which qualify as the follows:

1. A preload is included in the study

2. Adequate data on the energy intake of the test meal and preloads are provided.

3. The subjects are screened adequately for eating behaviours or circumstances that might affect their responses to the test such as:

a. individuals who were dieting, taking medication, pregnant or breastfeeding

b. dietary restraint

c. eating disorder

d. depression

e. eating attitude

f. they like the food to be served

4. Measurements are likely to be valid and reliable.

5. Steps are taken to minimize placebo effects in conducting the test.

6. Sample size is justified and statistical significance is assessed

7. Numbers add up correctly and are consistent in the paper

8. The researches are examined whether the null findings are adequately explained and whether there are any important effects overlooked.

Studies rejected after the above screening have been noted and reasons tabulated. Studies on individual with eating disorder were not included in the data analysis below. Included were those for healthy individuals who are normal weight, lean, overweight or obese.

An initial 48 papers were found of which 32 research papers satisfied the following inclusion criteria:

• contain at least one preload in their study

• the subjects included healthy normal weight individuals or overweight and obese individuals with no eating disorders or restraint eating habits

• the study was conducted with the objectives of studying one of the effects listed in this section.

• The full research article can be found

116

These studies are as are listed in the References together with newer researches made for the purpose of creating this Book added.

V.   Data Analysis

Given that each research will have a different approach to its data analysis, one of the major tasks of the dissertation is to present the data in a way to facilitate comparison across researches. In order to facilitate this, the following data points will be extracted from the research studies:

1. Studies

2. Subjects

3. Preload Used

4. Macronutrient composition

5. Energy of Preload (kJ)

6. Volume (ml) or Weight (g)

7. Time before meal from preload start (mins)

8. Physical state of preload (solid, liquid, mix)

9. Preload energy as % of no preload meal

10. Meal Compensation (1)

11. Total ST (Short Term) Food Intake (2)

12. Total ST Meal Compensation (32)

13. Significant Differences between preloads and control and different groups if there are more than one group studied (43)

The following computation and denotation will be used for parameters 9-13, 10 and 11 above:

(1) computed as energy of the test meal with preload as a percentage of the no preload test meal

(2) computed as the preload energy plus the food energy intake during the test meal

(3) computed as total energy of the preload and test meal as a percentage of the no preload test meal

(4) different letters are used in the tables and charts to indicate significant difference between food energy intake measures under different preload conditions within the respective studies. For example if two energy intake value is marked by the letter 'a', then this indicates that these two outcomes were found to have no significant difference. If an energy intake value is marked by 'a' and 'b', then there was significant difference found between these two outcomes.

The control is taken to be the meal without preload. If the control in the study is not a meal without preload, either a close and justifiable alternative is used, for example a control with preload of water. If the data is not available for any particular column, a 'na' is used.

In most of the preload conditions studied, there are usually more than one study found. Consistencies of the results of the studies will be examined and if there are differences in the results and conclusions, then these differences have to be examined and explained.

The parameters as listed above are summarized and tabulated.

The data in parameter 121, Total Short Term Meal Compensation, is examined to determine whether the preload can effectively reduce the total energy intake of both preload and the main meal. If it is less than 100%, then it indicates that for that test conditions, it has effectively reduced overall energy intake.

Each of the effects as listed below is examined, studied and explained:

1. Optimal macronutrient composition

2. Optimal energy level

3. Optimal volume/weight composition

4. Optimal time effect

5. Preferred physical state of preload

6. Behavioural differences with different subject groups.

The total meal compensation will be graphically plotted against each of the parameters above for analysis. For macronutrients, it will be plotted against the percentage composition of each of the macronutrients to examine for optimal level. The Total Short Term food intake which represents the preload calorie plus the food intake at test meal is plotted against each of the variables 1-6 above to examine for the effects of

118

the parameter on the food energy intake and whether compensation is observed. The significant difference is also taken into account.

A conclusion can draw on the implications of the reviews relating to the initial hypothesis that it sets out to examine. Constraints encountered in the review are noted, for example, if only abstract is available and not the full article etc.

VI.   Limitations

The limitation of this dissertation study was that it is dependent on researches already published and the availability of these articles from either online or at the public and university libraries in Singapore (where I was located at the time of the dissertation) or whether the authors were contactable if the articles could not be located online and at the university libraries.

Out of the 32 preload researches found, three did not publish the energy intake information of the test meal, one did not publish the relevant energy intake data, one is a review of previous studies on sugar preloads and the full article could not be found for one.

Researches which did not publish the energy intake during the test meal or did not measure the intake include:

•   Yeomans, Lee and Gray, 2001

•   Spiegel et al, 1993

•   Lappalainen et al, 1993

•   Van de Ven et al, 1994

Van de Ven et al (1994) did not published the data for the 30 min interval test where significant difference was found in the subsequent food intake for the test meal after the high fructose-high fibre preload compared to a placebo.   But instead, they provided the data for the 60 min when no such significant difference was found. So, the data were not compiled but the article would be used for references.

In one case, only abstracts can be found and the full articles are not available. In such cases, the researches will be listed for information. After all efforts, Rodin (1990) could not be located as the article was too old and there was no author contact information available.   The study was on the comparative effects of fructose, aspartame, glucose and water on calorie and macronutrient intake. However, this article had been cited by Anderson and Woodend (2003) and Rolls (1999) and these articles were found and included amongst the preload studies.

Out of these preload studies, energy intake data can only be extracted from 27 of the studies and the rest of the studies are used as references for qualitative comparison.

In some researches, the total day energy was also measured to examine whether the effects of the preload lingered onto the rest of the day but in some, this was not measured.

Appendix B: Common Foods & Approximate Calories per 100g

The tables below reveal the approximate energy of everyday foods—empowering you to craft your own nourishing, balanced, pre-meal recipes with confidence and creativity. The 100g indicated below is pre-cook weight.

Animal-based Proteins	Calories (kcal/100g)	Energy (kJ/100g)
White meat:		
Chicken breast (skinless)	120	502
Fish, non-fatty (cod)	82	343
Fish, non-fatty (tilapia)	96	402
Fish, salmon	208	871
Prawns (without shell)	71	297
Turkey breast	111	464
Red meat:		
Beef (lean)	187	782
Duck (lean, skinless)	140	586
Lamb (lean)	206	862
Pork (lean)	143	598
Venison (lean)	158	661

Dairy:		
Cheese, Brie	334	1398
Cheese, Camembert	300	1255
Cheese, Cheddar	402	1681
Cheese, Colby	402	1681
Cheese, Cottage	98	410
Cheese, Edam	357	1494
Cheese, Mozzarella	280	1172
Yogurt, unsweetened low-fat	63	264
Yogurt, standard (whole milk/plain)	97	406
Milk, standard	62 per 100 ml	260 per 100ml
Milk, low-fat	46 per 100 ml	260 per 100ml

Egg Size (USA / NZ)	Weight (approx.)	Calories (kcal /egg)	Energy (kJ / egg)
Jumbo / 9	70 g	90	377
Extra-Large / 8	63 g	80	335
Large / 7	56 g	72	301
Medium / 6	49 g	63	264
Egg White	100 g	52 per 100g	218

Plant-based Proteins (pre-cook weight)	Protein (g/100g)	Calories (kcal / 100g)	Energy (kJ / 100g)
Almonds	21	576	2411
Black Beans	9	339	1419
Cashews	18	553	2314
Chia Seeds	17	486	2034
Chickpeas	9	164	686
Edamame	11	122	511
Green Peas	5	81	339
Hemp Seeds	31	553	2314
Hummus	7	166	695
Kidney Beans	9	333	1394
Lentils	9	116	486
Lima Beans	7	113	473
Long Beans	1.6	47	197
Peas (Green)	5	81	339
Pine Nuts	14	673	2816
Quinoa	8	120	502
Seitan (wheat gluten)	25	370	1548
Soy Milk	3	45	188
Spelt	15	338	1414
Tempeh	19	192	803
Tofu	8	76	318

Non-starchy vegetables	Calories (kcal / 100g)	Energy (kJ / 100g)
Broccoli	34	142
Button Mushrooms	22	92
Cabbage	25	105
Capsicums (Bell Peppers)	20	84
Carrots	41	172
Cauliflower	25	105
Celery	16	67
Courgettes (Zucchini)	17	71
Cucumber	15	63
Eggplant (Aubergine)	25	105
Lettuce	15	63
Long Beans	47	197
Mung Bean Sprouts	30	126
Onions	40	167
Radish	16	67
Spinach	23	96
Tomatoes	18	75

Fruits	Calories (kcal / 100g)	Energy (kJ / 100g)
Apples	52	218
Apricots	48	201
Bananas	89	372
Blackberries	43	180
Blueberries	57	238
Feijoas	55	230
Grapes, green	69	289
Grapes, red	69	289
Honeydew melon	36	151
Kiwifruits, gold	60	251
Kiwifruits, green	61	255
Nectarines	44	184
Oranges	47	197
Pears	57	238
Pears, Nashi	42	176
Pineapple	50	209
Plums	46	192
Pomegranate Arils	83	347
Raspberries	52	218
Rock melon	34	142
Strawberries	32	134
Watermelon	30	126

Appendix C: Common Foods & Approximate Calories per oz

The tables below reveal the approximate energy content of everyday foods—empowering you to craft your own nourishing, balanced, pre-meal recipes with confidence and creativity.

Animal-based Protein (pre-cook)	Calories per oz
White meat:	
Chicken breast (skinless)	34.0
Fish, non-fatty (cod)	23.2
Fish, non-fatty (tilapia)	27.2
Fish, salmon	59.0
Prawns (without shell)	20.1
Turkey breast	31.5
Red meat:	
Beef (lean)	53.0
Duck (lean, skinless)	40.0
Lamb (lean)	58.4
Pork (lean)	41.0
Venison (lean)	44.8

Dairy:	
Cheese, Brie	94.7
Cheese, Camembert	85.1
Cheese, Cheddar	114.0
Cheese, Colby	114.0
Cheese, Cottage	27.8
Cheese, Edam	101.2
Cheese, Mozzarella	79.4
Yogurt, Greek	17.9
Yogurt, unsweetened low-fat	17.9
Yogurt, standard (whole milk/plain)	27.5
Milk, standard (1 US fl oz)	19.0
Milk, low-fat (1 US fl oz)	13.0

Egg Size (USA / NZ)	Weight (oz)	Calories (per egg)
Jumbo / 9	2.5	100
Extra-Large / 8	2.3	90
Large / 7	2.0	80
Medium / 6	1.8	70
Egg White (per 100g)	3.5	52

Plant-based Protein	Protein (g per oz pre-cook)	Calories (per oz pre-cook)
Almonds	6.0	163.3
Black Beans	2.6	96.1
Cashews	5.1	156.8
Chia Seeds	4.8	137.8
Chickpeas	2.6	46.5
Edamame	3.1	34.6
Green Peas	1.4	23.0
Greek Yogurt (dairy)	2.8	17.9
Hemp Seeds	8.8	156.8
Hummus	2.0	47.1
Kidney Beans	2.6	94.4
Lentils	2.6	32.9
Lima Beans	2.0	32.0
Long Beans	0.5	13.3
Peas (Green)	1.4	23.0
Pine Nuts	4.0	190.8
Quinoa	2.3	34.0
Seitan	7.1	104.9
Soy Milk	0.9	12.8
Spelt	4.3	95.8
Tempeh	5.4	54.4
Tofu	2.3	21.5

Non-starchy vegetables	Calories per oz
Aubergine (Eggplant)	7.1
Broccoli	9.6
Button Mushrooms	6.2
Cabbage	7.1
Capsicums (Bell Peppers)	5.7
Carrots	11.6
Cauliflower	7.1
Celery	4.5
Cucumber	4.3
Lettuce	4.3
Long Beans	13.3
Mung Bean Sprouts	8.5
Onions	11.3
Radish	4.5
Spinach	6.5
Tomatoes	5.1
Zucchini (Courgettes)	4.8

Fruits	Calories per oz
Apples	14.7
Apricots	13.6
Bananas	25.2
Blackberries	12.2
Blueberries	16.2
Feijoas	15.6
Grapes, green	19.6
Grapes, red	19.6
Honeydew melon	10.2
Kiwifruits, gold	17.0
Kiwifruits, green	17.3
Nectarines	12.5
Oranges	13.3
Pears	16.2
Pears, Nashi	11.9
Pineapple	14.2
Plums	13.0
Pomegranate Arils	23.5
Raspberries	14.7
Rock melon	9.6
Strawberries	9.1
Watermelon	8.5

Appendix D: Plant-based protein (g) to match 50g of chicken breast meat in calories (~82 kcal)

Plant-based Food (pre-cook)	Calories per 100g Pre-Cook	Estimated Pre-Cook Weight (g)
Almonds	579.0	14.2
Black Beans	369.6	22.2
Cashews	553.0	14.8
Chia Seeds	486.0	16.9
Chickpeas	459.2	17.9
Edamame	145.2	56.5
Green Peas	100.8	81.3
Hemp Seeds	553.0	14.8
Hummus	166.0	49.4
Kidney Beans	355.6	23.1
Lentils	324.8	25.3
Lima Beans	322.0	25.5
Long Beans	47.0	174.5
Peas (Green)	100.8	81.3
Pine Nuts	673.0	12.2
Quinoa	336.0	24.4
Seitan (wheat gluten)	370.0	22.2
Soy Milk (unsweetened)	33.0	248.5
Spelt	355.6	23.1
Tempeh	193.0	42.5
Tofu (firm)	144.0	56.9

Appendix E: Plant-based protein (oz) to match 50g of chicken breast meat in calories (~82 kcal)

Plant-based Food (pre-cook)	Calories per 1 oz Pre-Cook	Estimated Pre-Cook Weight (oz)
Almonds	164.1	0.5
Black Beans	104.8	0.78
Cashews	156.8	0.52
Chia Seeds	137.8	0.6
Chickpeas	130.2	0.63
Edamame	41.2	1.99
Green Peas	28.6	2.87
Hemp Seeds	156.8	0.52
Hummus	47.1	1.74
Kidney Beans	100.8	0.81
Lentils	92.1	0.89
Lima Beans	91.3	0.9
Long Beans	13.3	6.16
Peas (Green)	28.6	2.87
Pine Nuts	190.8	0.43
Quinoa	95.3	0.86
Seitan (wheat gluten)	104.9	0.78
Soy Milk (unsweetened)	9.4	8.77
Spelt	100.8	0.81
Tempeh	54.7	1.5
Tofu (firm)	40.8	2.01

About the Author

Hester Y Cheong: A Mind for Clarity, A Passion for Insight

Hester Cheong brings together scientific precision and a gift for clear communication. With a Master's degree in **Exercise and Nutrition Science from the University of Chester (UK)**—awarded with **Distinction**—she transforms complex research into practical, impactful strategies that support real-world health outcomes. The foundation of this Book grew from her dissertation on **preloads and appetite regulation**, which earned her the Distinction award and now forms the core of this reader-friendly guide.

Hester is endlessly curious and empirically driven. Whether she is dissecting the mechanisms of satiety, exploring the metabolic effects of food timing, or translating a dense research paper into accessible guidance, she does so with integrity and purpose.

Beyond academia, Hester served as a **project manager for a weight loss programme** with the New Zealand Research Institute for Plant and Food Research, applying scientific insights to real people, in real situations. She does not just study nutrition—she **questions it, tests it, and reimagines it** to help others achieve lasting change.

Whether refining the tone of a metabolic study or meticulously calculating the calories in a seafood soup, Hester combines intellect with heart. No shortcuts. No hype. Just clarity, curiosity, and a deep commitment to empowering others through science.